MIND DIET

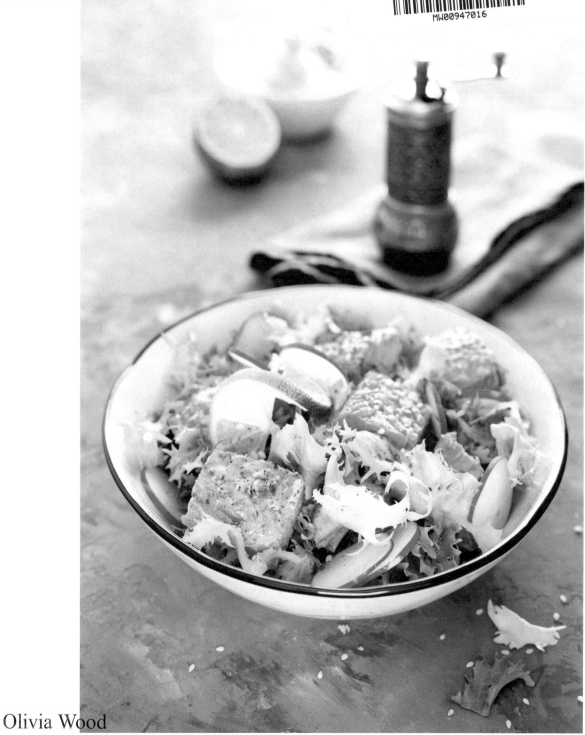

Olivia Wood

LEGAL & DISCLAIMER

The information contained in this book and its contents is not designed to replace or take the place of any form of medical or professional advice; and is not meant to replace the need for independent medical, financial, legal, or other professional advice or services, as may be required. The content and information in this book has been provided for educational and entertainment purposes only.

The content and information contained in this book has been compiled from sources deemed reliable, and it is accurate to the best of the Author's knowledge, information, and belief. However, the Author cannot guarantee its accuracy and validity and cannot be held liable for any errors and/or omissions. Further, changes are periodically made to this book as and when needed. Where appropriate and/or necessary, you must consult a professional (including but not limited to your doctor, attorney, financial advisor, or such other professional advisor) before using any of the suggested remedies, techniques, or information in this book.

Upon using the contents and information contained in this book, you agree to hold harmless the Author from and against any damages, costs, and expenses, including any legal fees potentially resulting from the application of any of the information provided by this book. This disclaimer applies to any loss, damages or injury caused by the use and application, whether directly or indirectly, of any advice or information presented, whether for breach of contract, tort, negligence, personal injury, criminal intent, or under any other cause of action. You agree to accept all risks of using the information presented inside this book.

You agree that by continuing to read this book, where appropriate and/or necessary, you shall consult a professional (including but not limited to your doctor, attorney, or financial advisor or such other advisor as needed) before using any of the suggested remedies, techniques, or information in this book.

2

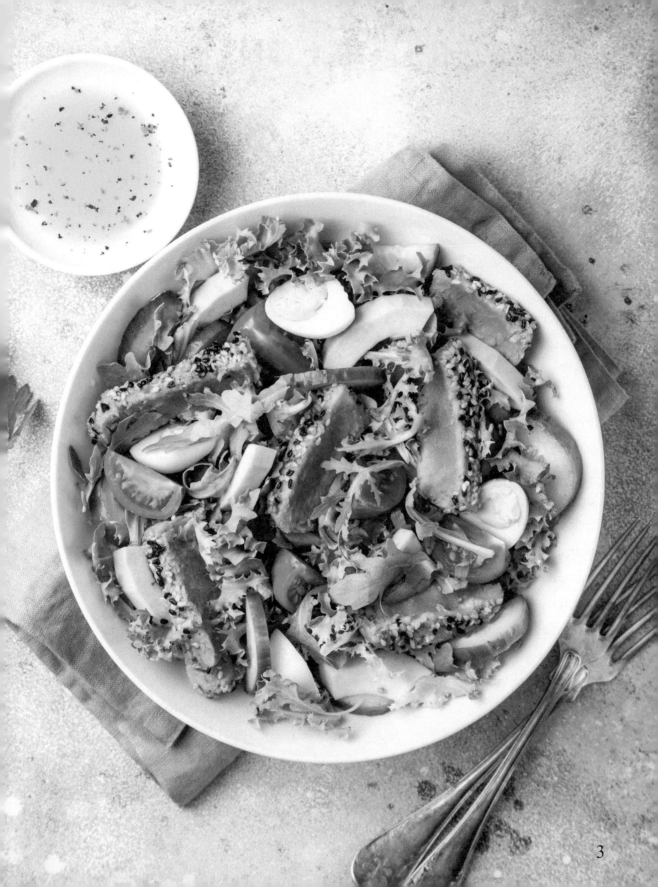

TABLE OF CONTENTS

INTRODUCTION 6

WHAT IS THE MIND DIET 8

MIND DIET SUITABLE FOODS 13

FOODS YOU SHOULD AVOID 18

WHAT LIFESTYLE SHOULD
YOU ADOPT TO REDUCE
YOUR RISK OF ALZHEIMER'S 22

BREAKFAST RECIPES 28

Sage Zucchini Cakes 30

Chia Pudding 32

Sweet Potato Noodles With
Hollandaise Sauce 34

Spinach And Eggs Salad 36

Vegetable Sandwich 37

Carrot Apple Smoothie 38

Chili Tomatoes And Eggs 40

Salmon And Green Onion Omelette 42

Blueberry & Mint Parfaits 44

Delicious Quinoa & Dried Fruit 46

Turmeric Scramble 48

Bean Pate 49

Chickpea Cookie Dough 50

Banana Pancakes 52

Mushroom Omelet 54

Peaches And Cream 56

MAIN DISHES 58

Salmon Teriyaki 60

Delightful Coconut Vegetarian
Curry 62

Thyme Chicken Mix 64

Coconut Veggie Wraps 66

Spinach And Mashed Tofu Salad 68

Cucumber Edamame Salad 70

Garlic Calamari Mix 72

Chili Cod 73

Five Spice Chicken Breast 74

Quinoa Edamame Salad 76

Apple Lentil Salad 78

Sweet Potato And White Bean
Skillet 80

Green Beans And Potatoes 82

Chickpea And Spinach Cutlets 84

Chili Collard Greens 86

Coconut Chickpea Curry 88

Balsamic-Glazed Roasted
Cauliflower 90

Garlicky Kale & Pea Sauté 92

Salad With Avocado 93

Black Bean Stuffed Sweet Potatoes 94

Salmon And Potato Salad 96

Tasty Roast Salmon 98

Coriander Shrimp Salad 100

Roasted Cod With Bok Choy 102

Salmon Cutlets 104

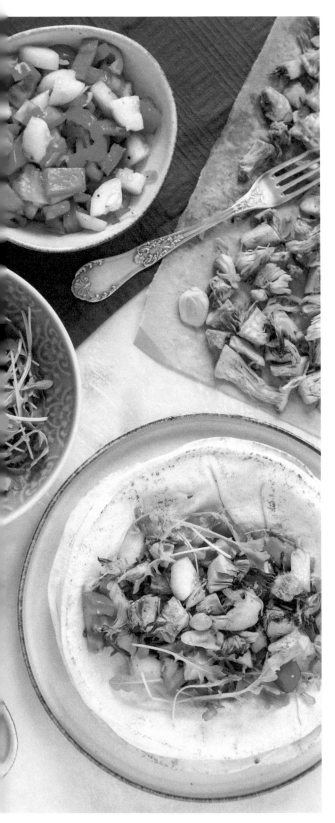

Shrimp Salad	106
Salmon And Shrimp Bowls	107
Cheesy Turkey Pan	108
Turkey And Endives Salad	110
Chicken Salad	111
Chicken Pieces	112
Baked Chicken With Sweet Paprika	114
Mandarin Chicken Stir Fry	116
Shrimp And Asparagus Salad	118
Roasted Chicken Breast And Vegetables	120
SNACKS & DESSERTS	122
Chocolate Peanut Butter Energy Bites	124
Potato Chips	126
Beets Chips	127
Lentils Spread	128
Rosemary And Sweet Potato Chips	130
Rainbow Fruit Salad	132
Almonds And Seeds Bowls	134
Roasted Walnuts	135
Cranberry Squares	136
CONCLUSION	138

INTRODUCTION

In the realm of health, few conditions evoke as much concern and fear as Alzheimer's disease. Widely perceived as an affliction of the elderly, the stereotypical image often centers on memory loss. However, the reality is more nuanced and significantly more challenging. Confronting a diagnosis of Alzheimer's or dementia poses a formidable struggle for both the affected individual and their family.

Alzheimer's disease stands as the predominant form of dementia, a formidable brain disorder with profound implications for daily living. Unfurling as a tapestry of memory loss and cognitive shifts, its impact reverberates throughout the individual's life. Notably, the Alzheimer's Association emphasizes that not every instance of memory loss equates to Alzheimer's, yet statistics reveal its pervasive reach. One in ten individuals over the age of sixty-five, and almost one-third of those surpassing eighty-five, grapple with this formidable condition. The insidious onset of Alzheimer's unfolds gradually, its symptoms evolving and intensifying over time. Commencing with inconspicuous forgetfulness, it burgeons into pervasive brain impairment as critical cells succumb, culminating in the stark loss of personality and systemic failure. Self-diagnosis proves elusive, necessitating prompt medical attention when signs become conspicuous.

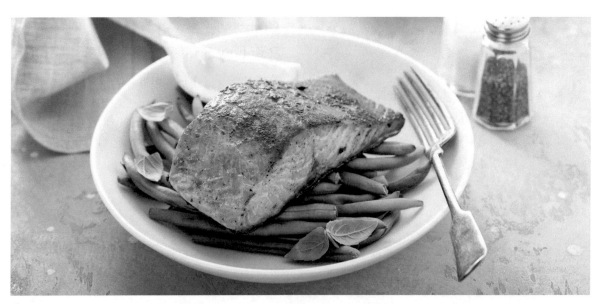

While fear may accompany the prospect of diagnosis, early intervention and assistance afford a greater opportunity to stave off debilitating symptoms. Appropriate medical intervention not only extends autonomy but optimizes the quality of life.

Despite Alzheimer's prevalence and its seeming inevitability with aging, there exists a realm of proactive measures for prevention. Fundamental among these is the profound influence of diet and lifestyle. Many remain unaware that daily choices in nutrition and habits carry enduring implications for long-term health, even in those seemingly in the pink of health.

This book is crafted with a singular purpose — to unravel the manifold benefits of the MIND diet. Each chapter meticulously navigates critical facets, from the development and diagnosis of Alzheimer's to the specific dietary recommendations endorsed by the MIND diet and lifestyle modifications essential for reducing the risk of this formidable disease.

The underlying premise of this book is empowerment — empowering you with the knowledge to preemptively safeguard against Alzheimer's and dementia through transformative alterations in dietary and lifestyle choices. In any facet of life, information is paramount. Swift access to the necessary insights enables proactive measures, mitigating potential harm. It is never too early to reshape your life, cultivating habits that may become the cornerstone of a serene and healthy existence in your golden years.

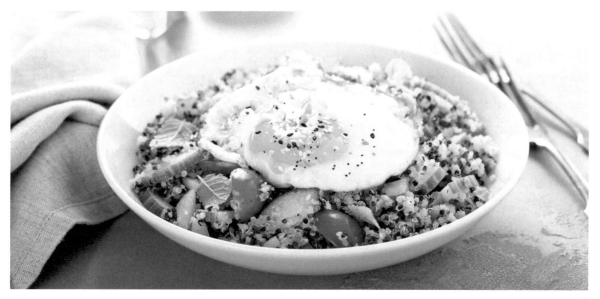

WHAT IS THE MIND DIET

You've likely encountered the age-old adage, «you are what you eat.» These words of wisdom, echoed even by healthcare professionals, underscore the profound influence of our dietary choices on the intricate workings of the brain. Recent groundbreaking research conducted at Rush University Medical Center in Chicago unveils a tangible means of diminishing the risk of Alzheimer's disease through a specialized diet — the MIND diet. The staggering revelation from this study indicates a remarkable 53 percent reduction in Alzheimer's risk for those who embrace this dietary approach. Even individuals who don't strictly adhere to the MIND diet can significantly enhance their well-being, reducing the risk of this debilitating disease by one third.

Published in the esteemed journal Alzheimer's & Dementia, the study meticulously examined over nine hundred participants aged fifty-eight to ninety-eight. Through food questionnaires and repeated neurological testing, the results demonstrated that those aligning their diets with MIND recommendations exhibited cognitive function equivalent to a person 7.5 years younger.

The MIND diet ingeniously amalgamates key elements from two renowned nutritional paradigms — the Mediterranean diet and the DASH (Dietary Approaches to Stop Hypertension) diet. The name «MIND» itself is a fusion, representing the Mediterranean-DASH Intervention for Neurodegenerative Delay.

Diverging from its predecessors in crucial ways, the MIND diet has proven to be more effective in mitigating the risk of Alzheimer's. In our exploration, let's briefly delve into the Mediterranean diet, celebrated for its health benefits, encompassing healthy fats, omega-three fatty acids, and whole grains. Residents of Mediterranean countries, like Italy, France, Spain, Greece, and Croatia, are renowned for their slender figures and long, healthy lives, marked by a low risk of heart issues and other ailments.

The Mediterranean diet revolves around whole foods, excluding processed items, and features a rich array of fruits, vegetables, olive oil, fish, nuts, and a moderate intake of wine.

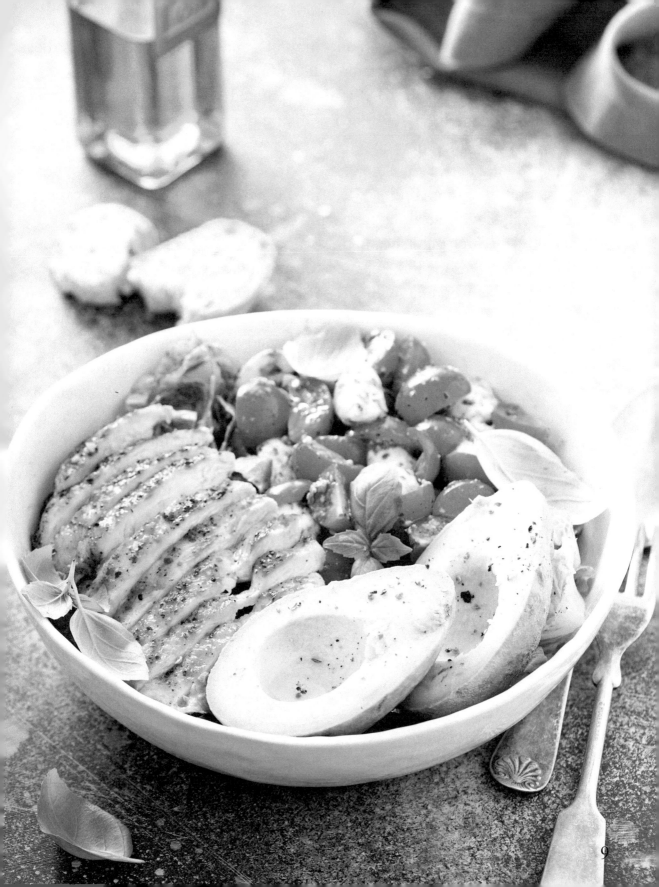

By cleansing the body of sugars, unhealthy fats, and processed foods, this diet diminishes the risk of high cholesterol, heart failures, and other diseases.

Turning our attention to the DASH diet, centered on fruits, vegetables, and low-fat dairy, it particularly excels in reducing the risk of stroke, heart attack, and hypertension. Incorporating flavonoid-rich produce into your diet, as suggested by a study in the Annals of Neurology, can potentially safeguard against cognitive aging. Fruits like strawberries and blueberries have been shown to delay cognitive aging in women by up to two and a half years.

Additionally, research published in the Journal of the Academy of Nutrition and Dietetics underscores the link between consuming leafy green vegetables, such as kale and spinach, and the reduction of inflammation and oxidative stress — factors associated with Alzheimer's disease. Foods rich in antioxidants play a crucial role in lowering inflammation and oxidative stress.

Oxidative stress, stemming from low antioxidant defenses and the body's inability to combat free radicals, has been implicated in various diseases, including cancer and Alzheimer's. The MIND diet focuses on plant-based foods while reducing the intake of animal products and saturated fats. In the upcoming chapter, we will delve into the specific foods essential for a proper MIND diet, unlocking the secrets to cognitive vitality and overall well-being.

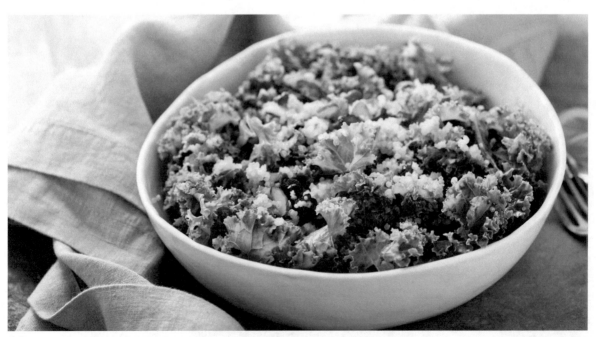

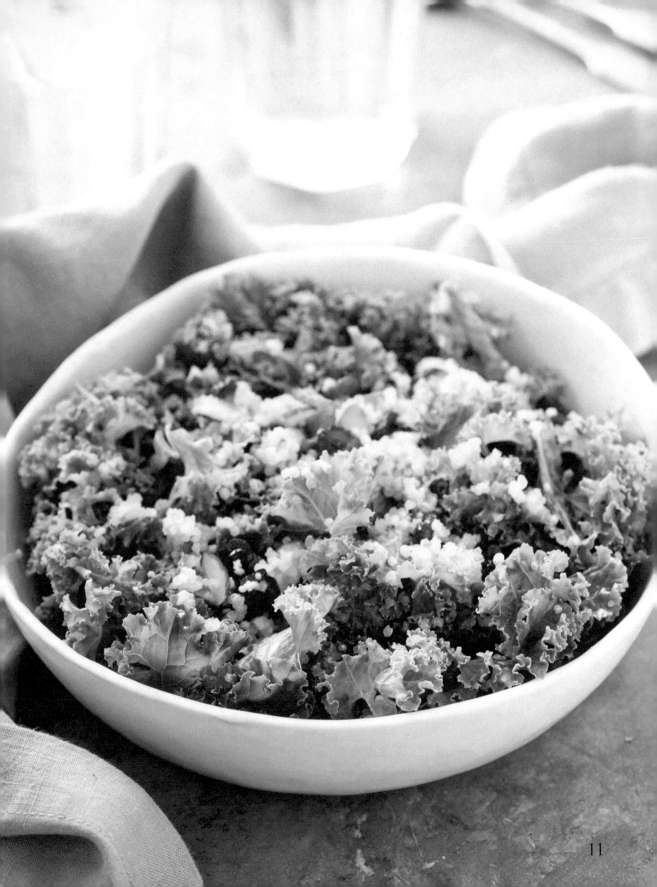

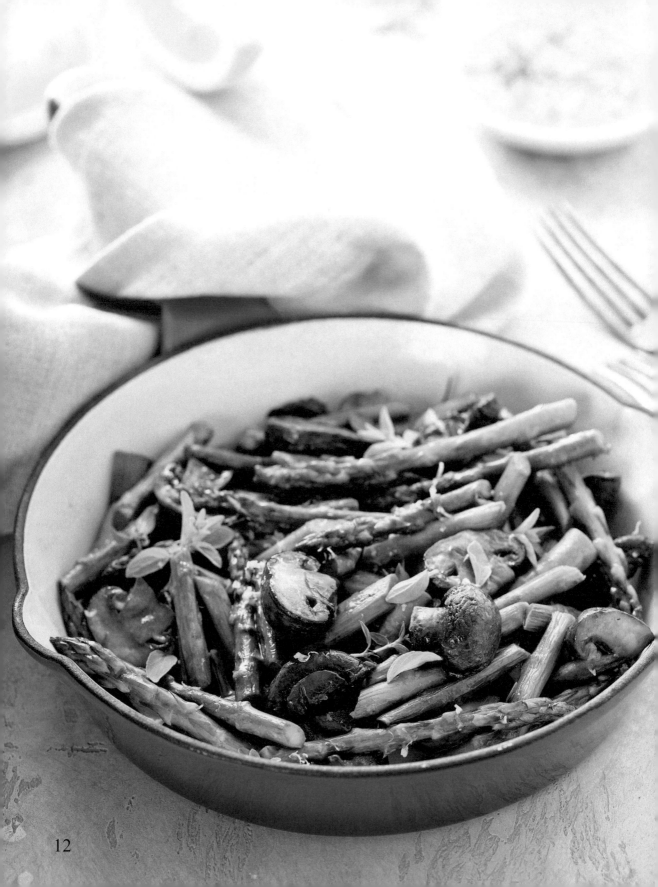

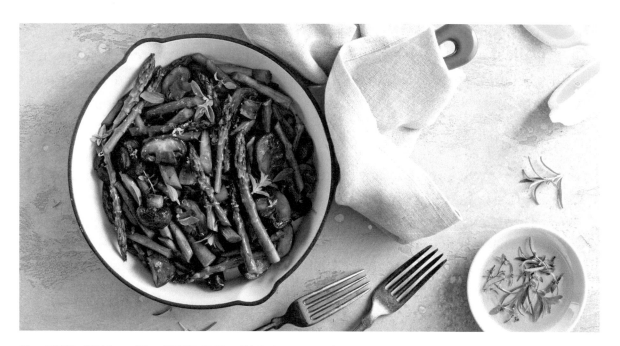

MIND DIET SUITABLE FOODS

Many individuals associate diets solely with weight loss or body detoxification, but it's crucial to recognize that not every diet serves the same purpose. Different dietary approaches yield various outcomes. As highlighted in the preceding chapters, the MIND diet is specifically designed to enhance brain health and act as a preventative measure against Alzheimer's disease.

As reiterated earlier, the MIND diet isn't exclusively tailored for those apprehensive about their Alzheimer's risk; it is beneficial for anyone seeking to maintain optimal brain function over the long term. Age is not a prerequisite to embark on this dietary journey. Whether you're in your twenties, thirties, or forties, embracing a regimen that includes fresh fruits and vegetables, minimizing or eliminating processed and junk foods, incorporating healthy fats, seafood, and reducing sugar, processed meat, and unhealthy fats can contribute significantly to sustaining cognitive well-being.

The subsequent sections will detail the foods well-suited for the MIND diet. It's important to note that weight concerns are not a prerequisite for adopting this dietary approach. The emphasis here lies on cultivating habits that foster a healthy and resilient brain, irrespective of one's weight status.

The cornerstone of the MIND diet lies in the abundance of fresh vegetables, with a particular emphasis on leafy greens. To kickstart your culinary journey, consider incorporating more frequent servings of nutrient-packed leafy greens such as spinach, kale, collards, broccoli, and other verdant vegetables. Rich in essential nutrients like vitamin A, vitamin C, and iron, these greens contribute to overall well-being.

If you're not accustomed to a vegetable-rich diet, take gradual steps towards integrating these nutritional powerhouses into your meals. Start by introducing a salad at least twice a week, although the recommendation is to include salads with every main meal of the day. Additionally, you can explore incorporating broccoli as a steamed side vegetable with your dinner, complementing dishes like poultry or pasta.

Researchers suggest that reaping optimal benefits involves consuming six or more servings of green vegetables per week. Notably, the MIND diet distinguishes itself from the DASH and Mediterranean diets, as it specifically underscores the impact of leafy green vegetables on reducing the risk of Alzheimer's.

The MIND diet underscores the pivotal role of vegetables in promoting brain health. Researchers recommend making a salad and consuming at least one vegetable every day as a proactive measure to mitigate the risk of Alzheimer's. In essence, embracing a vegetable-rich diet is not only a culinary choice but a strategic step towards safeguarding your cognitive well-being.

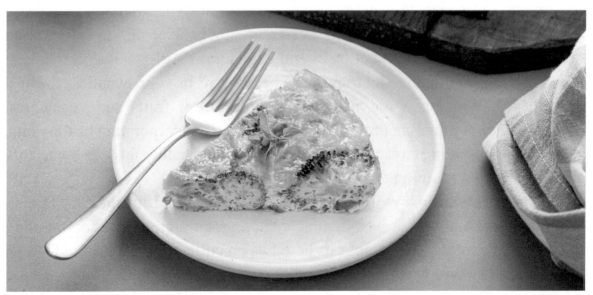

Moving along the MIND diet spectrum, nuts take center stage as delightful and nutritious snacks. Packed with healthy fats, antioxidants, and fiber, nuts offer a satisfying option to keep hunger at bay between meals. Research indicates that incorporating nuts into your diet can contribute to lowering bad cholesterol and reducing the risk of heart diseases. For MIND diet enthusiasts, it is recommended to enjoy nuts at least five times a week.

Shifting the spotlight to fruits, the MIND diet singles out berries as the preferred fruit category. While all berries are beneficial, blueberries emerge as particularly potent guardians of brain health. Strawberries also stand out, contributing to overall brain health and cognitive function. Including berries in your diet at least twice a week is not only a delightful addition to breakfasts but also a wholesome choice for healthy snacks.

Beans secure their place on the MIND diet roster as a nutritional powerhouse. Renowned for their high protein and fiber content, beans prove to be an excellent dietary component, catering to both vegans and vegetarians due to their low fat and calorie content. The MIND diet advocates for the inclusion of beans in your meals at least three times a week. Whether you're establishing a new habit or refining your existing choices, now is the opportune moment to embrace the brain-boosting benefits of beans.

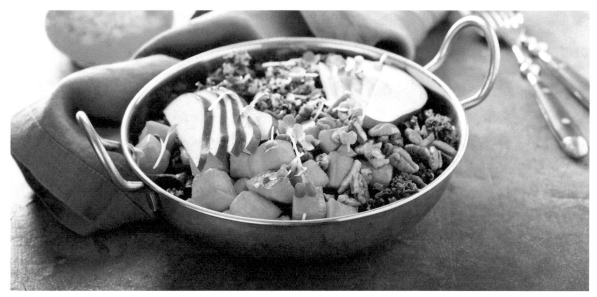

Becoming a doctor or nutritionist is not a prerequisite for understanding the importance of whole grains in maintaining a healthy diet. The MIND diet recommends a minimum of three servings of whole grains daily, emphasizing their integral role in supporting overall well-being.

For those concerned about the absence of meat in this dietary regimen, rest assured that the MIND diet incorporates fish into its recommendations. While fish is known to protect brain function, the diet suggests a moderate intake, advocating for its consumption at least once a week. This sets the MIND diet apart from the Mediterranean diet, which suggests a nearly daily consumption of fish.

Poultry also finds its place in the MIND diet as a means to foster long-term brain health. The diet recommends incorporating two or more servings of poultry into your weekly meals.

The manner in which you prepare your meals holds significance for any diet, and the MIND diet underscores the importance of cooking. Olive oil, renowned for its healthy fats, is the preferred choice for cooking. Research indicates that individuals who primarily use olive oil experience enhanced protection against cognitive decline.

Surprisingly, the MIND diet permits the inclusion of wine, allowing for a daily indulgence of one glass (not exceeding this limit). Celebrate the remarkable protective benefits of the MIND diet with a toast to your brain's well-being.

If certain foods within the MIND diet are unsuitable for you due to dietary restrictions (e.g., veganism, vegetarianism, allergies), there's no need to abandon the entire diet. Research suggests that even when followed moderately, the MIND diet continues to reduce the risk of Alzheimer's disease.

While this is a condensed list, it doesn't imply a restriction to these foods alone. Feel free to complement your weekly menu with a variety of other options, such as pasta, healthy desserts, Greek yogurt, and more. The key is to incorporate a diverse array of foods, with a focus on leafy greens, berries, fish, and olive oil, to maximize the benefits of the MIND diet.

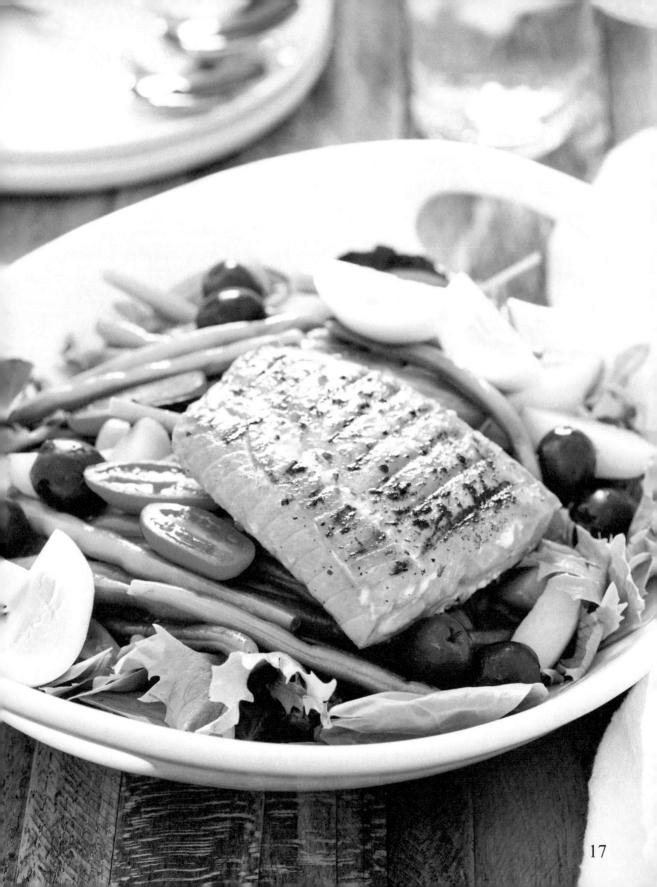

FOODS YOU SHOULD AVOID

In our journey to enhance cognitive vitality through the MIND diet, it's equally crucial to be mindful of the foods that might impede our brain health. While the MIND diet emphasizes the incorporation of brain-boosting foods, understanding what to limit or avoid is fundamental for comprehensive well-being.

Processed Foods

Processed foods, often laden with artificial additives, preservatives, and excessive salt, should be approached with caution. These items typically lack the nutritional value essential for optimal brain function. Steering clear of heavily processed snacks and meals supports the MIND diet's goal of nourishing the brain with wholesome, nutrient-rich choices.

Saturated Fats

Excessive intake of saturated fats, commonly found in red meat and full-fat dairy products, is linked to various health issues, including cardiovascular concerns. While the MIND diet doesn't eliminate meat entirely, it encourages moderation, emphasizing poultry over red meat to mitigate the potential negative impact on cognitive health.

Sugary Treats

A diet high in added sugars not only poses a risk to physical health but can also contribute to cognitive decline. Limiting the consumption of sugary treats, desserts, and sweetened beverages aligns with the MIND diet's emphasis on fostering a brain-friendly environment.

Trans Fats

Trans fats, commonly present in partially hydrogenated oils, have been associated with an increased risk of heart disease and cognitive impairment. The MIND diet advocates for steering clear of sources of trans fats, urging a preference for healthier cooking oils like olive oil.

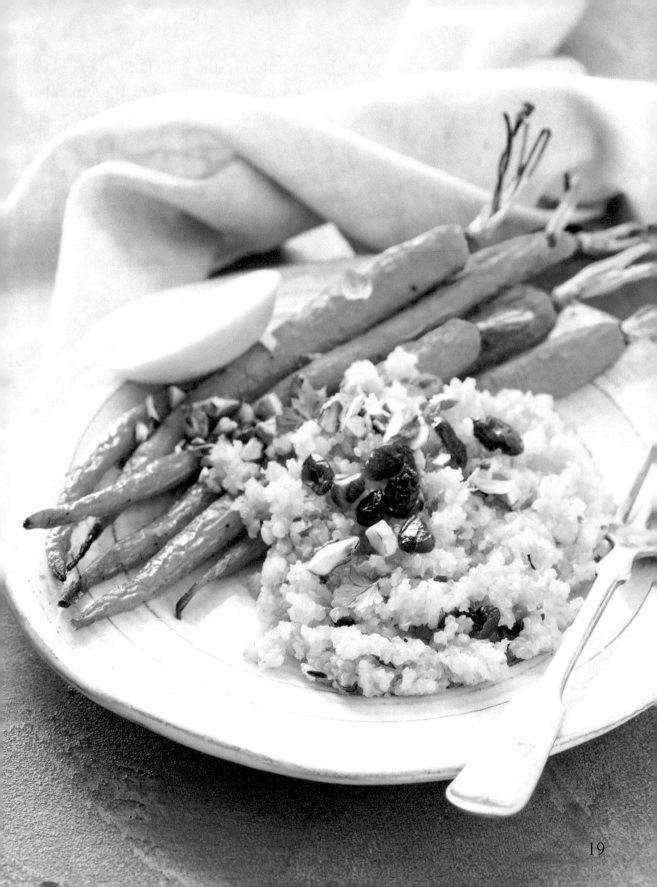

Excessive Alcohol

While moderate wine consumption is permitted in the MIND diet, excessive alcohol intake can have adverse effects on cognitive function. It's crucial to adhere to the recommended limit of one glass per day and refrain from exceeding this threshold.

High Sodium Foods

A diet rich in sodium can contribute to high blood pressure, which, in turn, may impact cognitive health. The MIND diet encourages the reduction of high-sodium foods, including processed snacks, canned soups, and certain condiments.

Limiting Dairy Intake

While dairy can be part of a balanced diet, excessive consumption of full-fat dairy products may introduce an undesirable amount of saturated fats. The MIND diet suggests moderating dairy intake and opting for low-fat or fat-free alternatives.

Understanding the foods to avoid is a complementary aspect of the MIND diet journey. By being mindful of processed foods, saturated fats, excessive sugars, trans fats, alcohol intake, high sodium foods, and dairy choices, you can create a dietary environment that maximizes the potential for long-term cognitive well-being.

What happens if you have a "cheat" day? It is entirely all right to reach for the foods that are not recommendable. You will still have benefits from the good foods if you consume them in larger amounts than the ones that are on this list. Researchers say that even if you are not following entirely this diet, you are still on the right track of reducing the risk for Alzheimer's disease. All you need to do is stick with this diet for a long time and get enough protection, a healthy functioning body, and good health.

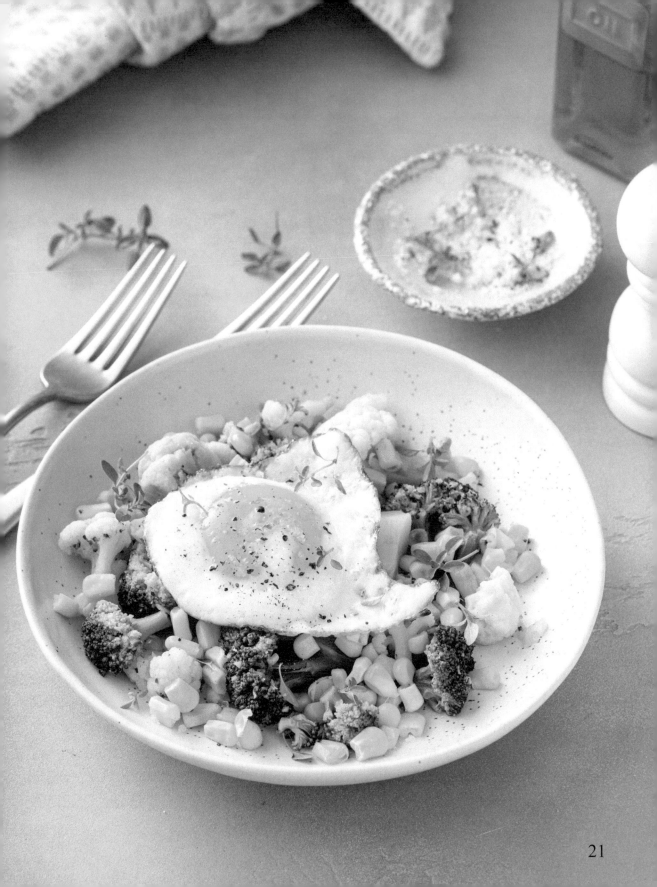

WHAT LIFESTYLE SHOULD YOU ADOPT TO REDUCE YOUR RISK OF ALZHEIMER'S

The MIND diet is more than just a meal plan; it's a comprehensive approach to brain health. To effectively reduce the risk of Alzheimer's, you must consider lifestyle factors that work in synergy with this diet. Let's explore how key habits can support cognitive health and strengthen the benefits of the MIND diet.

Regular Exercise
Physical activity is a critical component of brain health. Engaging in regular exercise improves blood flow to the brain, reduces inflammation, and promotes the growth of new neurons. Studies show that aerobic exercises like walking, swimming, and cycling are linked to a lower risk of cognitive decline. Exercise also enhances mood and energy levels, which are important for maintaining a positive and proactive approach to brain health. Coupled with the brain-boosting foods recommended by the MIND diet, regular physical activity can have a powerful impact on cognitive resilience.

Healthy Diet
While the MIND diet is specifically designed to protect the brain, adopting an overall healthy eating pattern reinforces its effects. Incorporating nutrient-rich foods, such as whole grains, fruits, vegetables, and lean proteins, supports not only brain function but overall body health. Prioritizing foods rich in antioxidants, omega-3 fatty acids, and vitamins can reduce inflammation and oxidative stress, both of which are linked to Alzheimer's disease. A balanced diet also supports vascular health, which is critical for optimal brain function.

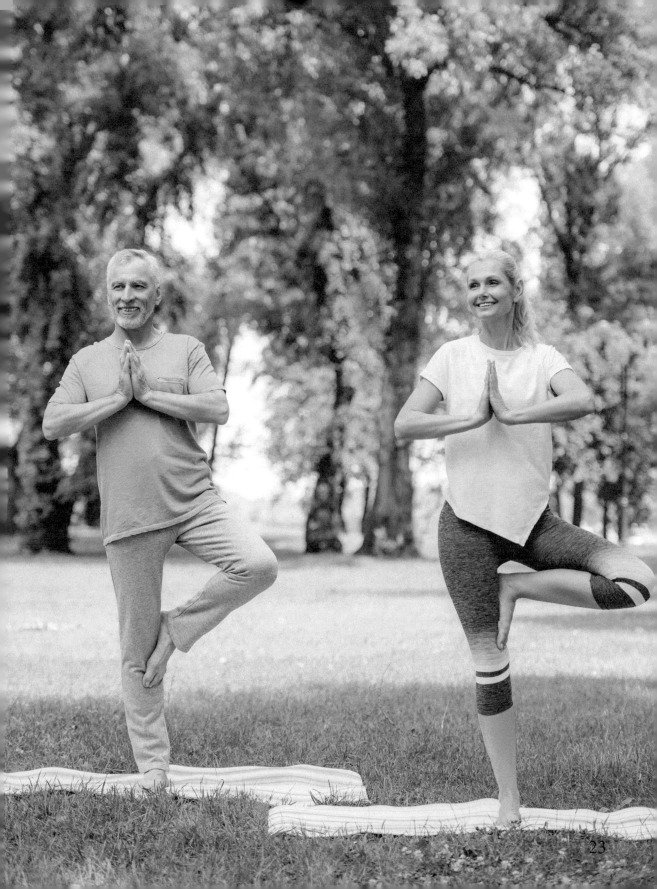

Social Engagement

Social interaction plays a vital role in maintaining brain health as we age. Engaging with family, friends, and communities helps to keep the mind active and stimulated. Isolation, on the other hand, is linked to a higher risk of cognitive decline. Participating in group activities or even simple daily conversations can improve memory retention, cognitive function, and mood, reducing the overall risk of Alzheimer's. Combining a socially active lifestyle with the MIND diet further enhances cognitive protection.

Mental Stimulation

Keeping the brain engaged through mental activities such as puzzles, reading, learning new skills, or playing instruments is essential for cognitive longevity. Mental stimulation promotes neuroplasticity, the brain's ability to reorganize itself by forming new neural connections. Regularly challenging your mind can prevent cognitive decline and lower the risk of Alzheimer's. The MIND diet provides the necessary nutrients to fuel brain activity, but it's important to pair it with mental exercises to achieve the best results.

Quality Sleep

Sleep plays a crucial role in maintaining brain health, as it is during deep sleep that the brain clears away waste products, including beta-amyloid plaques linked to Alzheimer's disease. Poor sleep can lead to memory problems and increase the risk of cognitive decline. Prioritizing consistent, quality sleep supports overall brain function and reinforces the neuroprotective effects of the MIND diet. Incorporating foods that promote better sleep, such as those rich in magnesium and melatonin, can further improve sleep quality.

Stress Management

Chronic stress negatively impacts brain health, increasing the risk of Alzheimer's through inflammation and hormonal imbalances. Prolonged stress can impair memory, cognitive function, and mood. Effective stress management techniques like meditation, deep breathing, or yoga can counteract these effects. Reducing stress, in combination with a diet that nourishes the brain, such as the MIND diet, creates a holistic approach to protecting cognitive health.

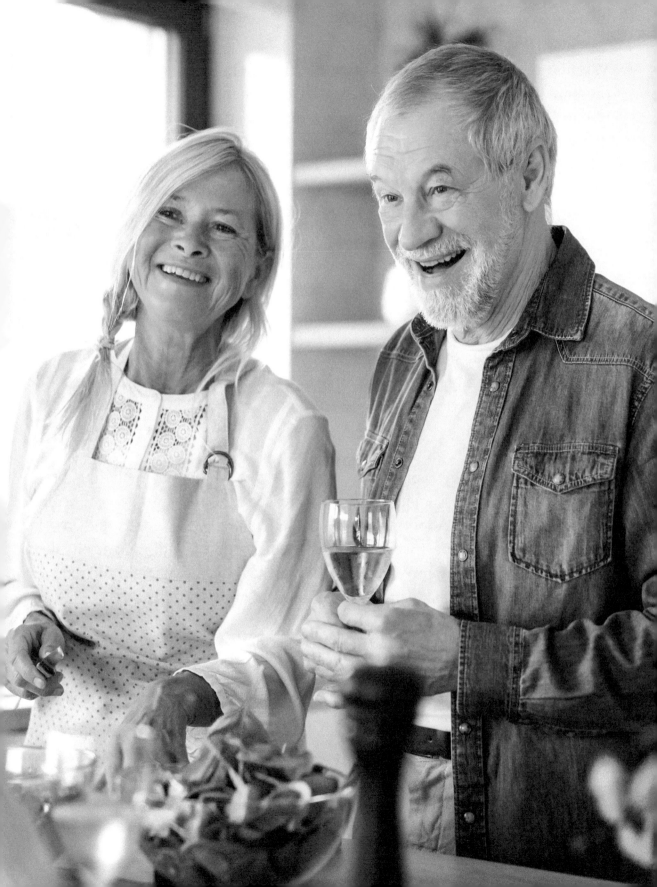

Vascular Health

Vascular health is closely tied to brain health. Conditions such as high blood pressure, high cholesterol, and diabetes can damage blood vessels, reducing blood flow to the brain and increasing the risk of Alzheimer's. The MIND diet emphasizes foods that protect the heart and blood vessels, such as leafy greens, nuts, and fish high in omega-3s. Maintaining a healthy heart supports cognitive function, as a strong cardiovascular system ensures the brain receives the oxygen and nutrients it needs to stay healthy.

Stay Hydrated

Proper hydration is often overlooked, but it's essential for maintaining optimal brain function. Dehydration can impair cognitive abilities and increase the risk of confusion and memory issues. Aim to drink adequate water throughout the day and incorporate hydrating foods, like fruits and vegetables, into your diet. A well-hydrated body supports brain health, making it an important aspect of the MIND diet lifestyle.

Healthy Weight Management

Maintaining a healthy weight is crucial for overall health, including brain function. Obesity is associated with an increased risk of cognitive decline and Alzheimer's disease. Adopting a MIND diet rich in whole foods and low in saturated fats can support weight management. Coupled with regular physical activity, this balanced approach helps maintain healthy body weight and reduces the risk of conditions that can negatively impact brain health.

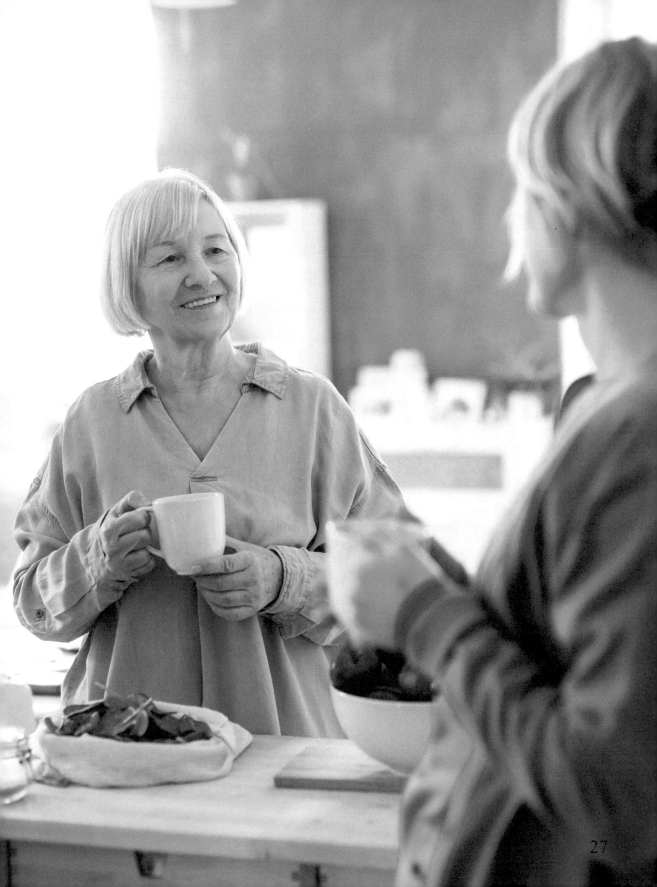

BREAKFAST RECIPES

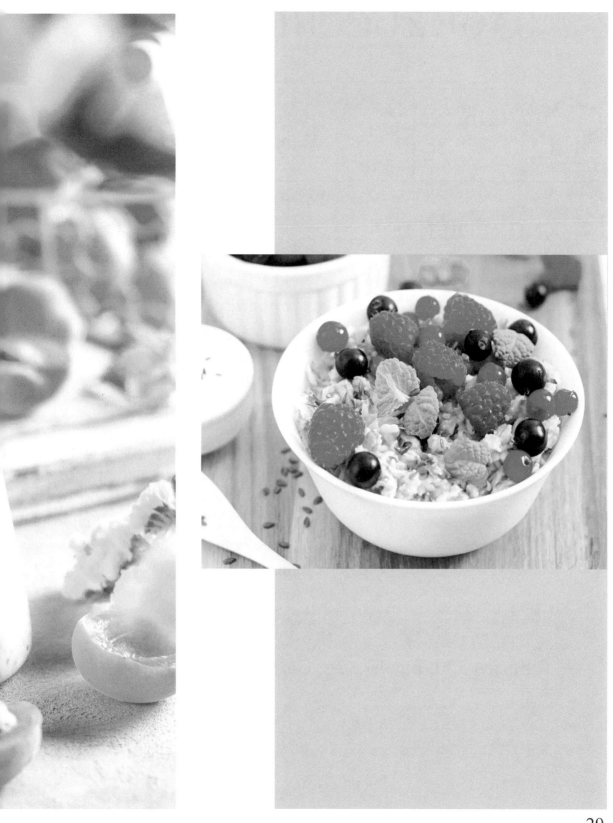

SAGE ZUCCHINI CAKES

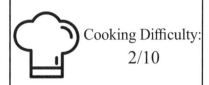 Cooking Difficulty: 2/10

 Cooking Time: 13 minutes

 Servings: 4

INGREDIENTS

- 1 lb. grated zucchinis, drained
- salt
- black pepper
- 1 tbsp. almond flour
- 1 whisked egg
- 1 tbsp. chopped sage
- 2 tbsps. olive oil

DESCRIPTION

STEP 1
In a bowl, combine the zucchinis with the flour and the other ingredients except for the oil, stir well and shape medium cakes out of this mix.

STEP 2
Ensure that you heat the pan, add the cakes, cook them for 5-6 minutes on each side, drain excess grease on paper towels, divide the cakes between plates and serve for breakfast.

NUTRITIONAL INFORMATION

Calories 320, Fat 13.32g, Carbs 10g, Protein 12.1g

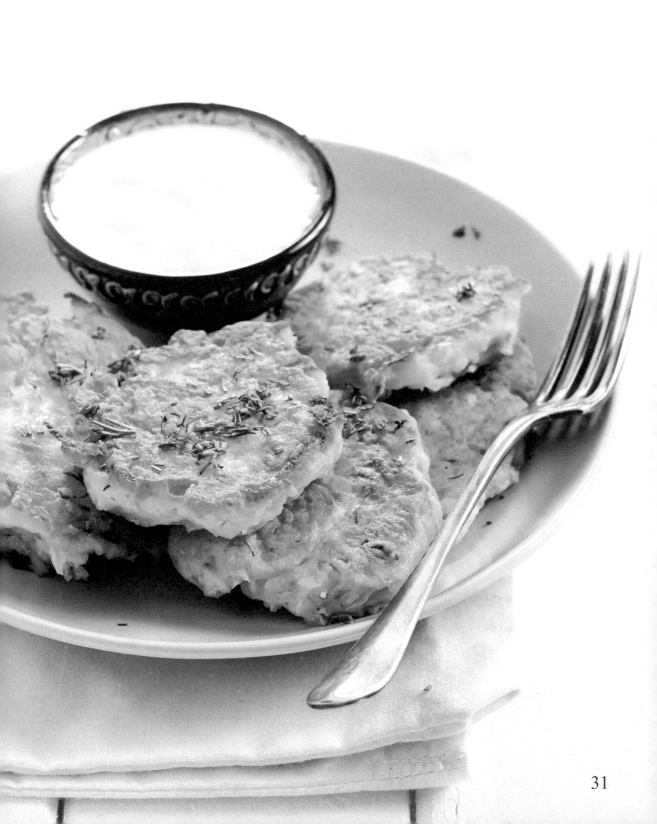

CHIA PUDDING

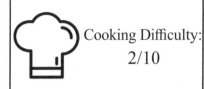 Cooking Difficulty: 2/10	Cooking Time: 32 minutes	Servings: 2

INGREDIENTS

- 1/3 c. coconut cream
- 55 g chia seeds
- 2 tbsps. cacao
- 1 tbsp. swerve
- 1 tbsp. vanilla sugar
- 2 c. water
- 2 tbsps. herbal coffee

DESCRIPTION

STEP 1
Brew the herbal coffee with some hot water until the liquid is reduced by half. Strain the coffee before mixing in with the vanilla, swerve, and coconut cream.

STEP 2
Add in the chia seeds and cacao nibs net. Pour into some cups and place in the fridge for 30 minutes before serving.

NUTRITIONAL INFORMATION

257 Calories, 20.25g Fats, 2.25g Net Carbs, 7gProtein

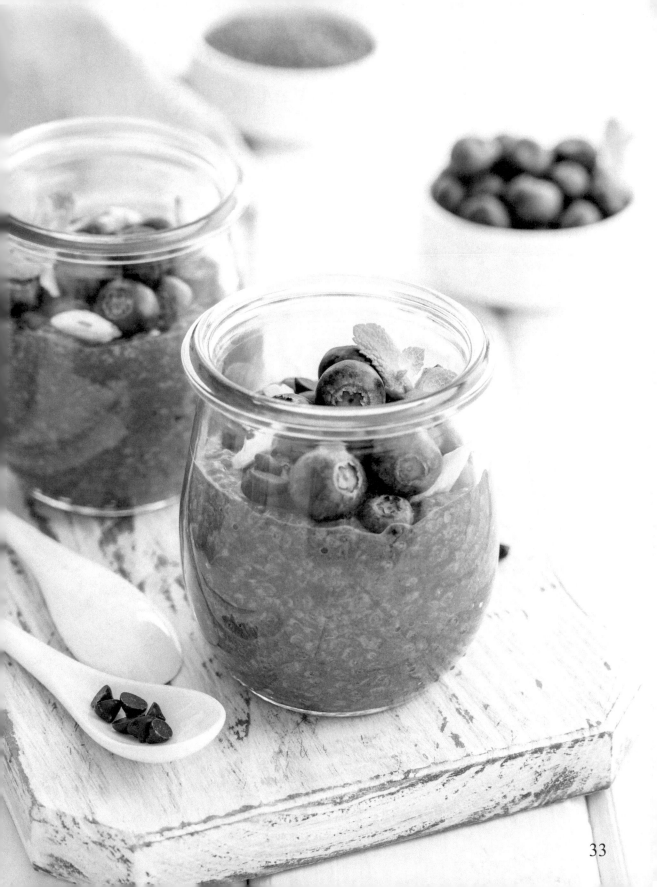

SWEET POTATO NOODLES WITH HOLLANDAISE SAUCE

 Cooking Difficulty: 4/10

 Cooking Time: 20 minutes

 Servings: 3

INGREDIENTS

- ¼ tsp. garlic powder
- 1 avocado, diced
- 1 trimmed sweet potato, noodles
- 1 tbsp. cilantro, chopped
- 3 eggs
- olive oil cooking spray
- black pepper
  for the sauce:
- 1 chipotle pepper
- 1 tsp. adobo sauce
- 1 tbsp. lemon juice
- 2 eggs yolks
- 3 tbsps. coconut oil, melted

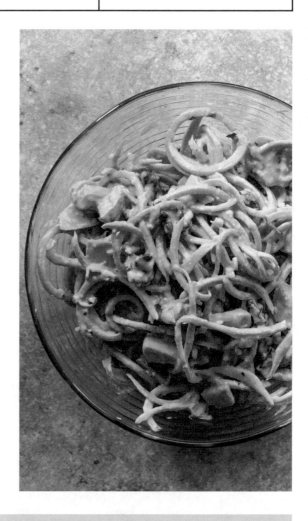

NUTRITIONAL INFORMATION

400 Calories, 33g Fat, 20g Carbs, 11g Protein

DESCRIPTION

STEP 1

Pre-heat your oven to 425 Degrees Fahrenheit. Lightly coat with cooking spray a baking sheet, place the sweet potato noodle and season it with pepper and garlic powder. Sprinkle avocado cubes on top and roast until the sweet potato noodles are cooked or for around 10 to 13 minutes.

STEP 2

Meanwhile, place the lemon juice, sauce, egg yolks, and chipotle pepper in a blender and pulse for around 10 seconds. Then, put the blender on medium and gradually add the coconut oil to thicken. Set aside. Once done with the hollandaise sauce, pour water in a medium saucepan fill it halfway and simmer.

STEP 3

Break the eggs into a small bowl or ramekin. Then, make a gentle whirlpool in the simmering water so the egg white will wrap around the yolk. Gradually tip the egg into the water. Cook for 3 mins. Remove eggs from water by use of a slotted spoon and transfer it on a paper towel-lined plate.

STEP 4

As soon as the avocado and sweet potato noodles are done, make a nest on 3 plates. Place poached eggs on top and drizzle with hollandaise sauce. Serve and garnish it with cilantro.

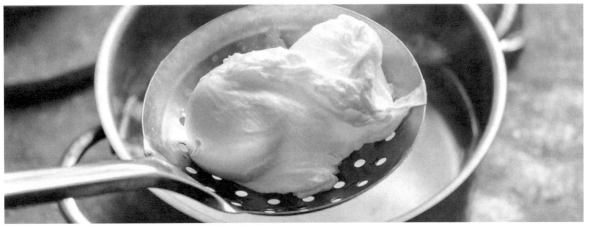

SPINACH AND EGGS SALAD

Cooking Difficulty: 2/10	Cooking Time: 3 minutes	Servings: 4

INGREDIENTS

- 2 c. baby spinach
- 1 c. cherry tomatoes
- 1 tbsp. chopped chives
- 4 peeled and cubed eggs
- salt
- black pepper
- 1 tbsp. lime juice
- 1 tbsp. olive oil

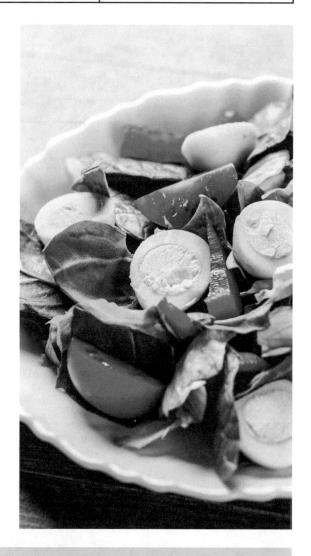

DESCRIPTION

STEP 1

In a bowl, combine the spinach with the tomatoes and the other ingredients, toss and serve for breakfast right away.

NUTRITIONAL INFORMATION

Calories 107, Fat 8g, Carbs 3.6g, Protein 6.4g

VEGETABLE SANDWICH

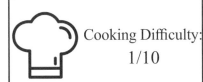 Cooking Difficulty: 1/10

 Cooking Time: 5 minutes

 Servings: 1

INGREDIENTS

- 2 pcs. whole-grain toast
- 2 tbsp. hummus
- ½ pcs. cucumber
- ½ pcs. avocado
- ¼ pcs. tomatoes
- 2 tbsp. grated carrots

DESCRIPTION

STEP 1

Toast the bread in a toaster. Cut the cucumber and tomato into slices, and cut the avocado into slices. Brush each toast with hummus. Place vegetables in random order on one slice of bread, top with another toast, and cut diagonally.

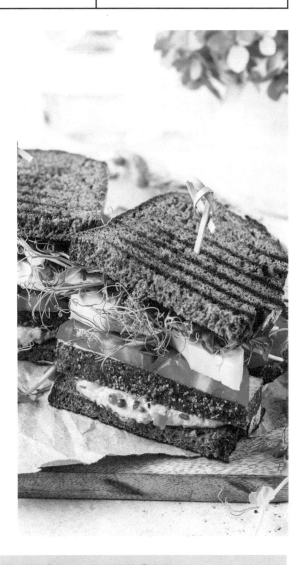

NUTRITIONAL INFORMATION

Calories: 336; Fat: 4.3 g; Carbs: 11.1 g; Protein: 4.6 g

CARROT APPLE SMOOTHIE

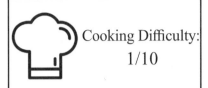 Cooking Difficulty: 1/10

 Cooking Time: 1 minutes

 Servings: 1

INGREDIENTS

- 2 c. baby spinach
- 1 medium apple, cored
- 1 tbsp. ginger, freshly grated
- 2 chopped carrots
- 1 c. filtered water

DESCRIPTION

STEP 1
Using a blender, set in all your ingredients until creamy and smooth. Serve right away!

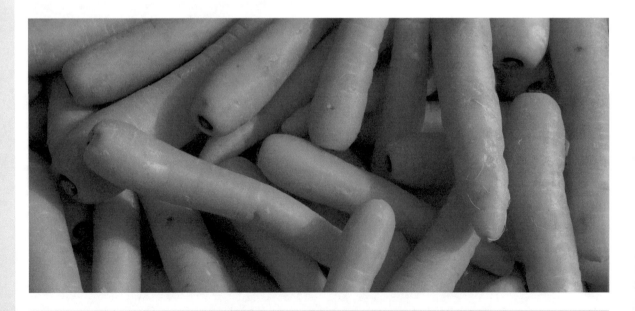

NUTRITIONAL INFORMATION

Calories 193, Fat 17.6 g, Carbs 8.3 g, Protein 2.3 g

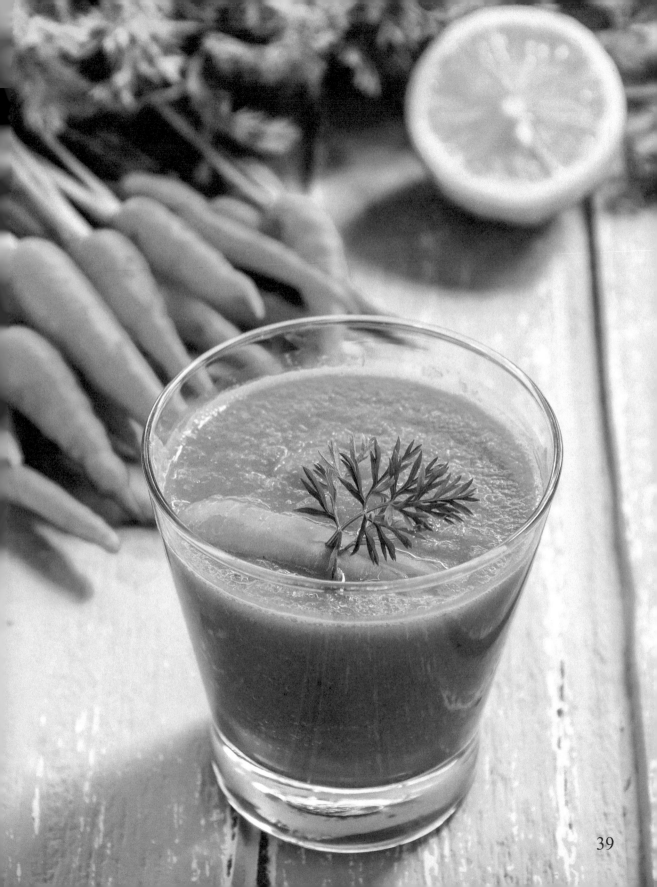

CHILI TOMATOES AND EGGS

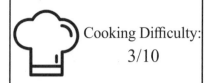 Cooking Difficulty: 3/10

 Cooking Time: 15 minutes

 Servings: 2

INGREDIENTS

- olive oil
- 2 chopped shallots
- 2 minced chili peppers
- salt
- black pepper
- 4 cubed tomatoes
- 4 whisked eggs
- 1 tsp. sweet paprika
- 1 tbsp. chopped chives

DESCRIPTION

STEP 1
Heat up a pan with the olive oil medium heat; add the shallots and the chili peppers, toss and sauté for 5 minutes.

STEP 2
Add the tomatoes and the other ingredients except for the eggs, toss, then cook everything for 5 minutes more.

STEP 3
Add the eggs, toss a bit, cook the mix for another 5 minutes, divide between plates and serve.

NUTRITIONAL INFORMATION

Calories 119, Fat 7.9g, Carbs 6.5g, Protein 6.9g

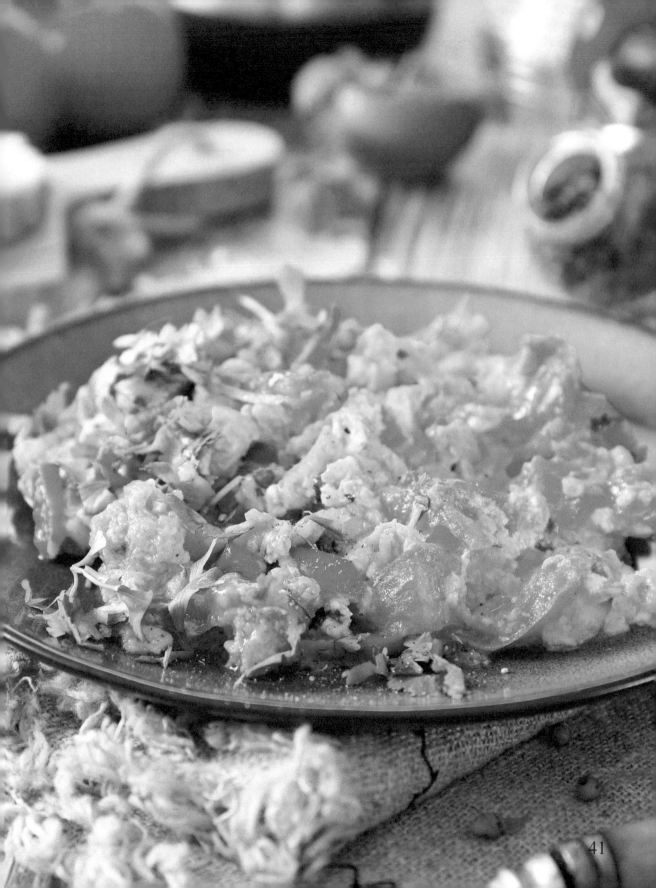

SALMON AND GREEN ONION OMELETTE

 Cooking Difficulty: 2/10

 Cooking Time: 6 minutes

 Servings: 1

INGREDIENTS

- 2 eggs
- 50g salmon (fried or boiled, diced)
- green onions (chopped)
- salt and pepper to taste
- 1 tablespoon olive oil

DESCRIPTION

STEP 1
Heat olive oil in a pan. Pour the beaten eggs into the pan. Add diced salmon and chopped green onions.

STEP 2
Season with salt and pepper to taste. Cook the omelette over medium heat until done.

NUTRITIONAL INFORMATION

25 Calories, 16g Fats, 20g Net Carbs, 3gProtein

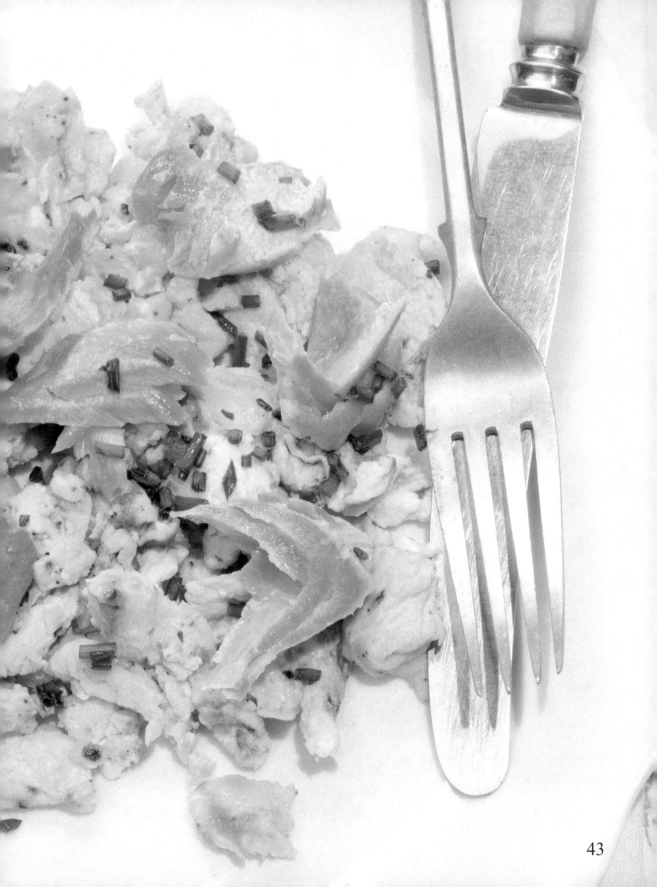

BLUEBERRY & MINT PARFAITS

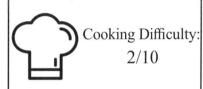 Cooking Difficulty: 2/10	Cooking Time: 5 minutes	Servings: 4

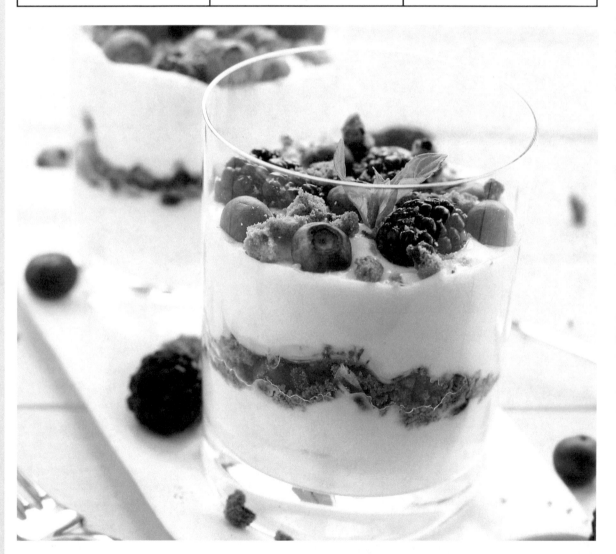

NUTRITIONAL INFORMATION

Calories: 272, Fat: 8g, Protein: 10g, Carbs: 25g

INGREDIENTS

- 1½ c. wholegrain rolled oats
- 1 c. almond milk
- 2 c. Greek yogurt, unsweetened
- 1 c. fresh blueberries
- blackberries (optional)
- 4 freshly chopped mint leaves

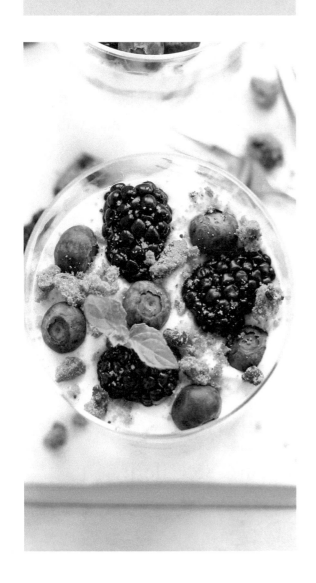

DESCRIPTION

STEP 1
Place the oats and almond milk into a bowl and stir together to combine (this helps the oats to soften).

STEP 2
Spoon the oat and almond milk mixture evenly into your 4 containers.

STEP 3
Place a drop of yogurt into each container on top of the oats (use half of the yogurt as you'll be adding another layer of it).

STEP 4
Divide half of the blueberries between the 4 containers and sprinkle on top of the yogurt.

STEP 5
Add another layer of yogurt and then another layer of blueberries (you can use them all up at this stage).

STEP 6
Sprinkle the fresh mint over the top of each parfait. Cover and place into the fridge to store until needed!

DELICIOUS QUINOA & DRIED FRUIT

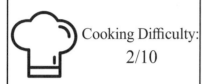 Cooking Difficulty: 2/10

 Cooking Time: 17 minutes

 Servings: 4

INGREDIENTS

- 3 c. water
- 1 c. quinoa
- ¼ c. cashew nut
- 8 dried apricots
- 4 dried figs
- 1 tsp. cinnamon

DESCRIPTION

STEP 1
In a pot, mix water and quinoa and let simmer for 15 minutes, until the water evaporates.

STEP 2
Chop dried fruit.

STEP 3
When quinoa is cooked, stir in all other ingredients.

STEP 4
Serve cold. Add milk, if desired.

NUTRITIONAL INFORMATION

44g Carbs, 7g Fat, 13g Protein, 285 Calories

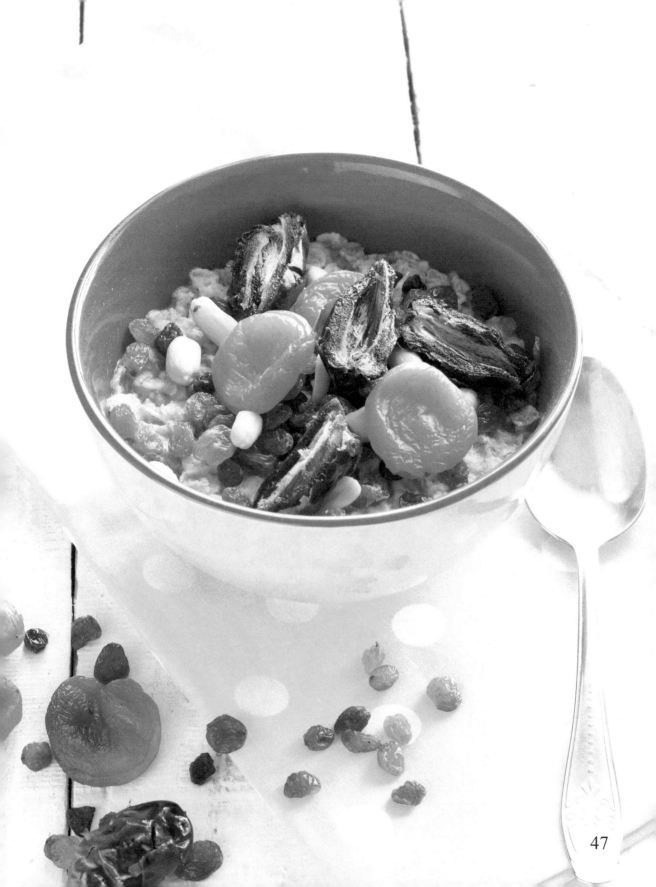

TURMERIC SCRAMBLE

 Cooking Difficulty: 3/10

 Cooking Time: 17 minutes

 Servings: 4

INGREDIENTS

- 1 tsp. turmeric powder
- 4 eggs, whisked
- 1 red bell pepper, chopped
- 2 shallots, chopped
- ¼ tsp. black pepper
- 1 tbsp. olive oil
- corn optional

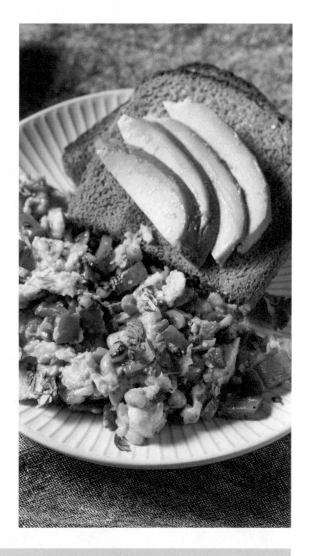

DESCRIPTION

STEP 1

Heat up a pan with the oil over medium heat, add the shallots and the bell pepper, stir and sauté for 5 minutes. Add the eggs mixed with the rest of the ingredients, stir, cook for 10 minutes, divide everything between plates and serve.

NUTRITIONAL INFORMATION

Calories 138, Fat 8g, Carbs 4.6g, Protein 12g

BEAN PATE

Cooking Difficulty: 2/10	Cooking Time: 10 minutes	Servings: 4

INGREDIENTS

- 1 cup cooked beans
- 1 onion
- ½ glass of water
- 1 pinch of salt
- olive oil

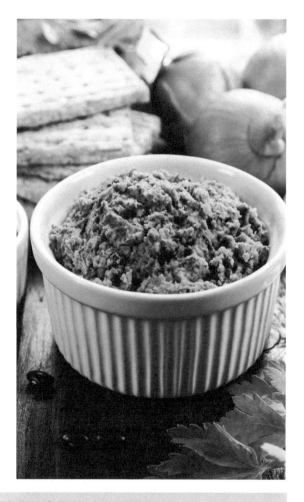

DESCRIPTION

STEP 1

Finely chop the onion and fry until translucent. Rinse the beans. Add oil and stir again. Combine the onion, beans, and spices in a blender. If the consistency is not uniform, add water or oil. Serve with whole-grain bread.

NUTRITIONAL INFORMATION

Calories: 160; Fat: 3.6 g; Carbs: 17.1 g; Protein: 6.1 g

CHICKPEA COOKIE DOUGH

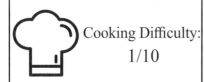 Cooking Difficulty: 1/10

 Cooking Time: 3 minutes

 Servings: 6

INGREDIENTS

- ½ tsp. sea salt
- 2 c. cooked chickpeas, drained
- ¼ c. maple syrup
- 1/3 c. melted coconut oil
- 3 tbsps. coconut flour
- 2 tsps. vanilla extract

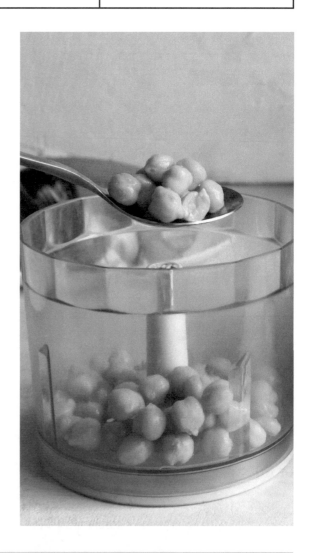

NUTRITIONAL INFORMATION

Calories: 415, Protein: 13.9g, Carbs: 54.4g, Fat: 16.9g

STEP 1

To make this delightful cookie dough, first, blend the chickpeas in a high-speed blender for a minute or until smooth.

STEP 2

Spoon in the oil, sea salt, maple syrup, and vanilla extract. Blend for a further minute or until combined.

STEP 3

Next, stir in the coconut flour and blend again. Scrape the sides.

STEP 4

Now, transfer the mixture to a medium-sized bowl and place in the refrigerator for 2 hours. Serve on its own or with crackers.

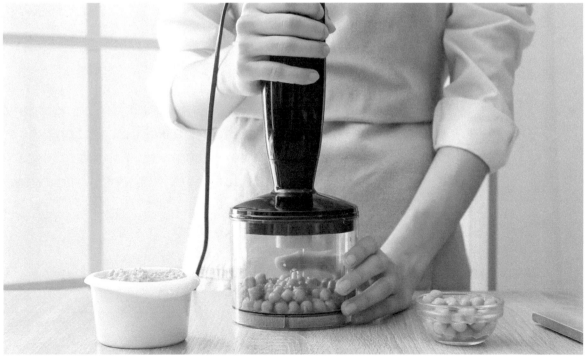

BANANA PANCAKES

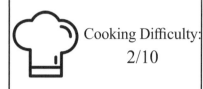 Cooking Difficulty: 2/10

 Cooking Time: 20 minutes

 Servings: 2

INGREDIENTS

- 2 bananas
- 1 egg
- ¼ glass of coconut milk
- 1 cup flour
- 1 teaspoon coconut oil

DESCRIPTION

STEP 1
Cut the bananas into pieces and place them in a blender along with an egg and a glass of milk (the milk should be warm).

STEP 2
Mix everything until smooth, and then gradually add flour, stirring constantly.

STEP 3
When the pancake dough is ready, heat the oil in a skillet. Spoon out the mixture and fry the pancakes on each side for about 30 seconds. Enjoy!

NUTRITIONAL INFORMATION

Calories: 210; Fat: 3.1 g; Carbs: 6g; Protein: 6.1 g

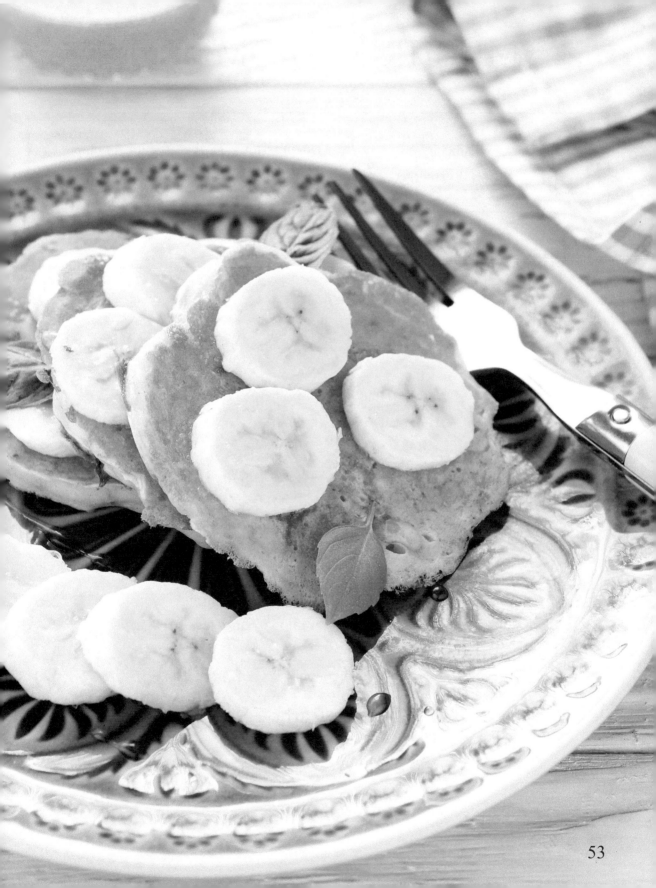

MUSHROOM OMELET

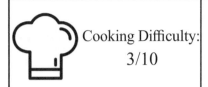 Cooking Difficulty: 3/10	Cooking Time: 15 minutes	Servings: 4

INGREDIENTS

- 2 chopped spring onions
- ½ lb. white mushrooms
- salt
- black pepper
- 4 whisked eggs
- 1 tbsp. olive oil
- ½ tsp. ground cumin
- 1 tbsp. chopped cilantro

DESCRIPTION

STEP 1
Ensure that you heat the pan; add the spring onions and the mushrooms, toss and sauté for 5 minutes.

STEP 2
Add the eggs and the rest of the ingredients toss gently, spread into the pan, cover it then cook over medium heat for 15 minutes.

STEP 3
Slice the omelet, divide it between plates, and serve for breakfast.

NUTRITIONAL INFORMATION

Calories 109, Fat 8.1g, Carbs 2.9g, Protein 7.5g

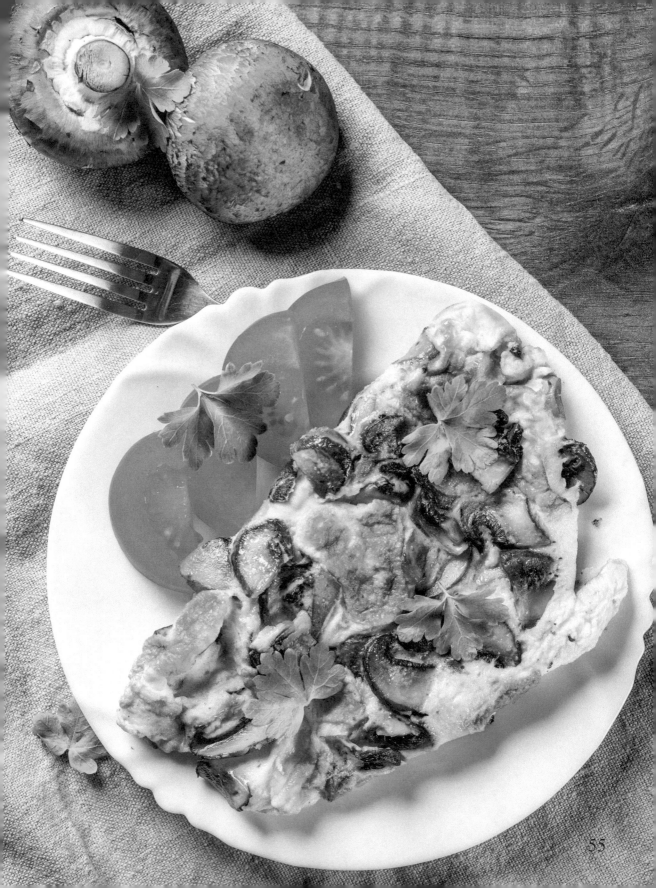

PEACHES AND CREAM

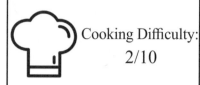 Cooking Difficulty: 2/10

 Cooking Time: 4 minutes

 Servings: 4

INGREDIENTS

- 2 c. coconut yogurt
- ½ c. water
- 1 pear, cored and chopped
- 2 tsps. pumpkin pie spice
- 2 tbsps. maple syrup
- ¼ c. cashews
- 2 c. pumpkin puree

DESCRIPTION

STEP 1

In a blender, combine the cashews with the water and the other ingredients except the yogurt and pulse well.

STEP 2

Divide the yogurt into bowls, also divide the pumpkin cream on top and serve.

NUTRITIONAL INFORMATION

Calories 200, Fat 6.4g, Carbs 32.9g, Protein 5.5g

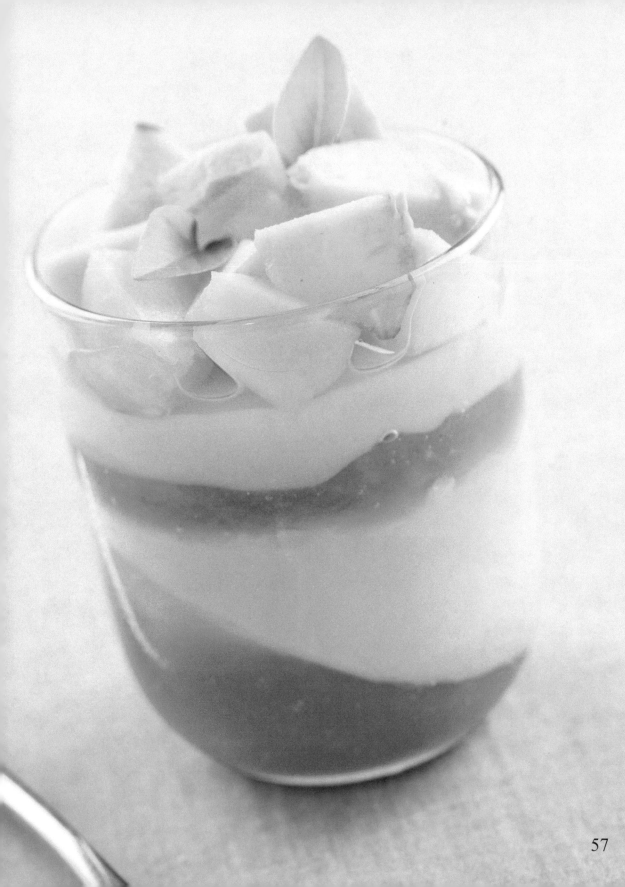

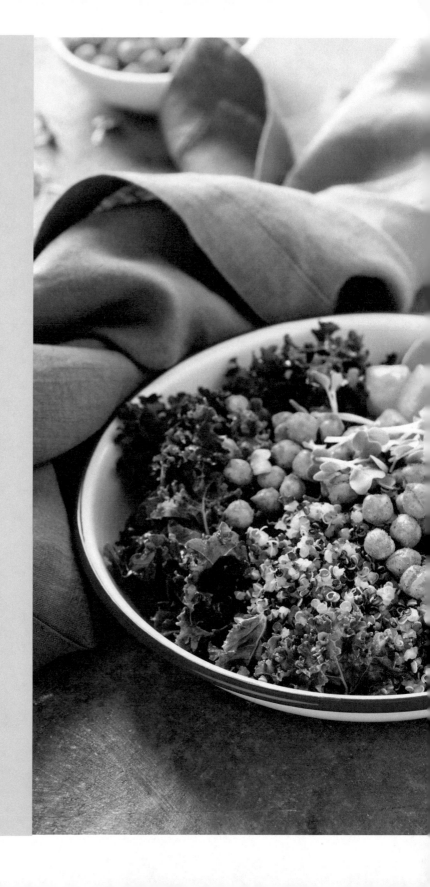

MAIN DISHES

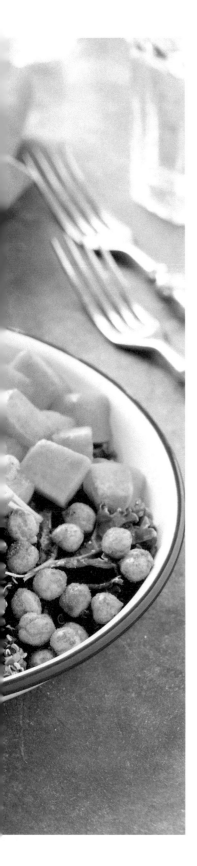

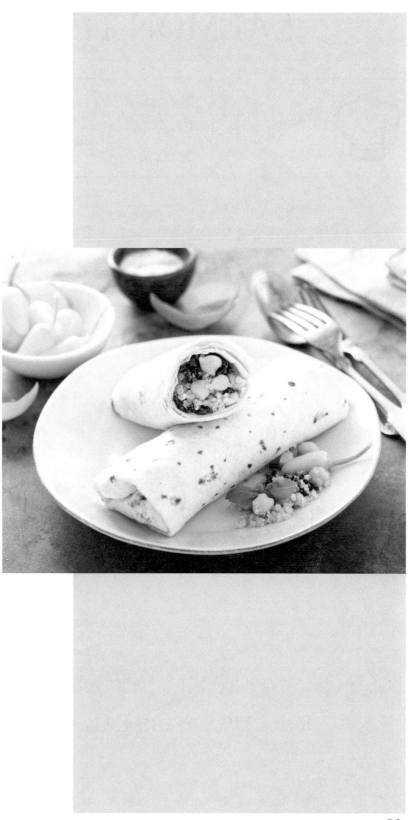

SALMON TERIYAKI

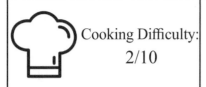 Cooking Difficulty: 2/10

 Cooking Time: 27 minutes

 Servings: 4

INGREDIENTS

- 6 tbsp. soy sauce
- 2 tbsp. chopped fresh ginger
- 2 tsp. minced garlic
- 4 salmon filet
- 2 tbsp. sesame seeds
- 1 lemon sliced thin

DESCRIPTION

STEP 1
Whisk together soy sauce ginger and garlic . Add optional sesame seeds if using.

STEP 2
Place salmon files in shallow dish and cover with soy-ginger sauce. Allow to marinate for 20 min.

STEP 3
Cover baking sheet with foil.Place fish on foil and top with any remaining marinade. Top with sliced lemon. Broil 5-7 min. Serve and enjoy!

NUTRITIONAL INFORMATION

Calories 279, Fat 18.7g, Carbs 9 g, Protein 24.1g

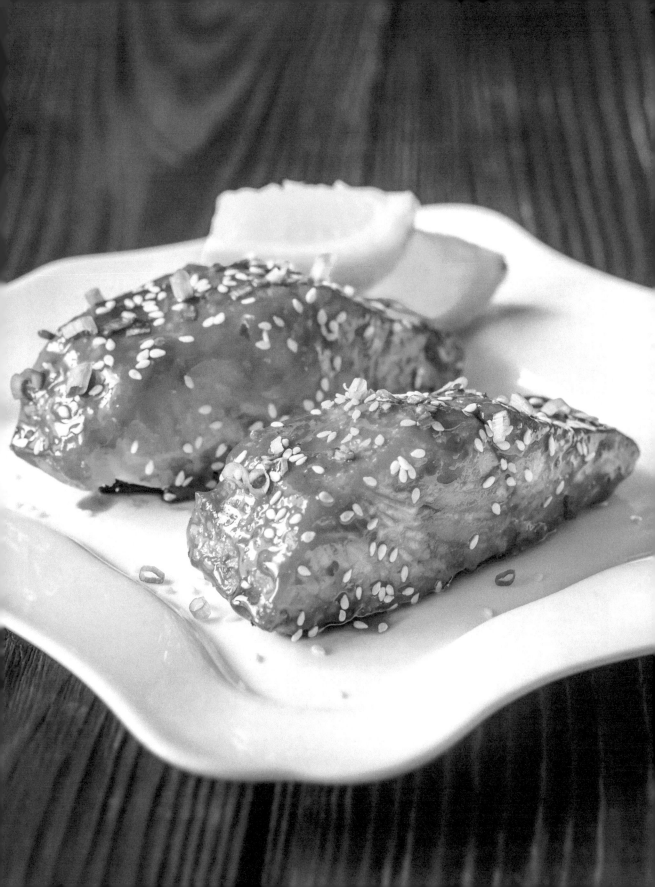

DELIGHTFUL COCONUT VEGETARIAN CURRY

Cooking Difficulty: 5/10	Cooking Time: 300 minutes	Servings: 6

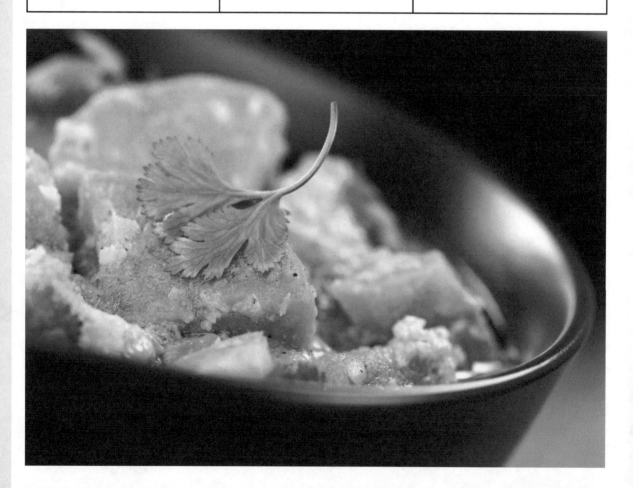

NUTRITIONAL INFORMATION

Calories:369 Cal, Carbs:39g, Protein:7g, Fats:23g

INGREDIENTS

- 5 potatoes, peeled and cubed
- ¼ c. curry powder
- 2 tbsps. flour
- 1 tbsp. chili powder
- ½ tsp. red pepper flakes
- ½ tsp. cayenne pepper
- 1 green bell pepper, chopped
- 1 red bell pepper, chopped
- 2 tbsps. onion soup mix
- 14 oz. coconut cream, unsweetened
- 3 c. vegetable broth
- 2 carrots, peeled and sliced
- 1 c. green peas
- ¼ c. chopped cilantro

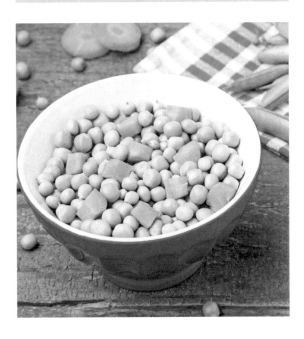

DESCRIPTION

STEP 1
Take a 6-quarts slow cooker, grease it with a non-stick cooking spray and place the potatoes pieces in the bottom.

STEP 2
Set in the rest of the ingredients except for peas, cilantro, and carrots.

STEP 3
Stir properly and cover the top.

STEP 4
Plug in the slow cooker; adjust the cooking time to 4 hours and let it cook on the low heat setting or until it cooks thoroughly.

STEP 5
When the cooking time is over, add the carrots to the curry and continue cooking for 30 minutes.

STEP 6
Stir in the peas to cook for 30 more minutes or until the peas get tender. Garnish it with cilantro and serve.

THYME CHICKEN MIX

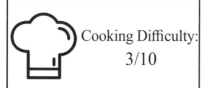 Cooking Difficulty: 3/10

 Cooking Time: 20 minutes

 Servings: 4

INGREDIENTS

- 1 lb. skinless and boneless chicken breast, sliced
- 1 tbsp. olive oil
- 2 chopped spring onions
- 1 c. baby spinach
- 1 tbsp. chopped thyme
- ½ c. tomato passata
- salt
- black pepper

DESCRIPTION

STEP 1
Ensure that you heat the pan, add the spring onions, and the meat and brown for 5 minutes.

STEP 2
Add the rest of the ingredients, bring to a simmer then cook over medium heat for 15 minutes, stirring from time to time.

STEP 3
Divide the mix into bowls and serve.

NUTRITIONAL INFORMATION

Calories 380, Fat 40g, Carbs 1g, Protein 17g

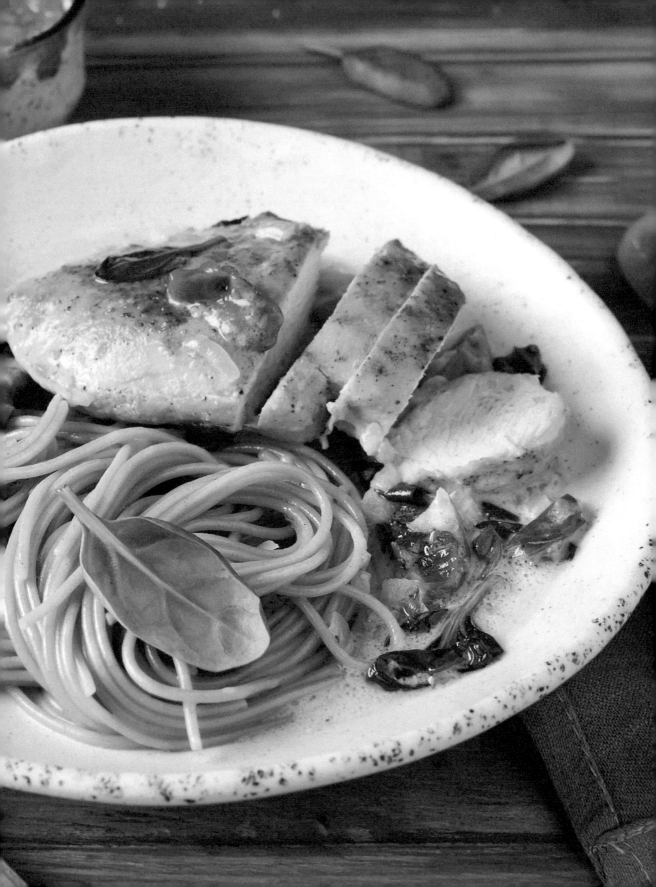

COCONUT VEGGIE WRAPS

 Cooking Difficulty:
3/10

 Cooking Time:
10 minutes

 Servings:
5

INGREDIENTS

- 1½ c. shredded carrots
- 1 red bell pepper, seeded, sliced
- 2½ c. kale
- 1 ripe avocado, sliced
- 1 c. fresh cilantro, chopped
- 5 coconut wraps
- 2/3 c. hummus
- 6½ c. green curry paste

DESCRIPTION

STEP 1
Slice, chop, and shred all the vegetables. Lay a coconut wrap on a clean flat surface and spread two tablespoons of the hummus and one tablespoon of the green curry paste on top of the end closest to you.

STEP 2
Place some carrots, bell pepper, kale, and cilantro on the wrap and start rolling it up, starting from the edge closest to you. Roll tightly and fold in the ends.

STEP 3
Place the wrap, seam down, on a plate to serve.

NUTRITIONAL INFORMATION

Calories 236, Carbs 23.6 g, Fats 14.3 g, Protein 5.5 g

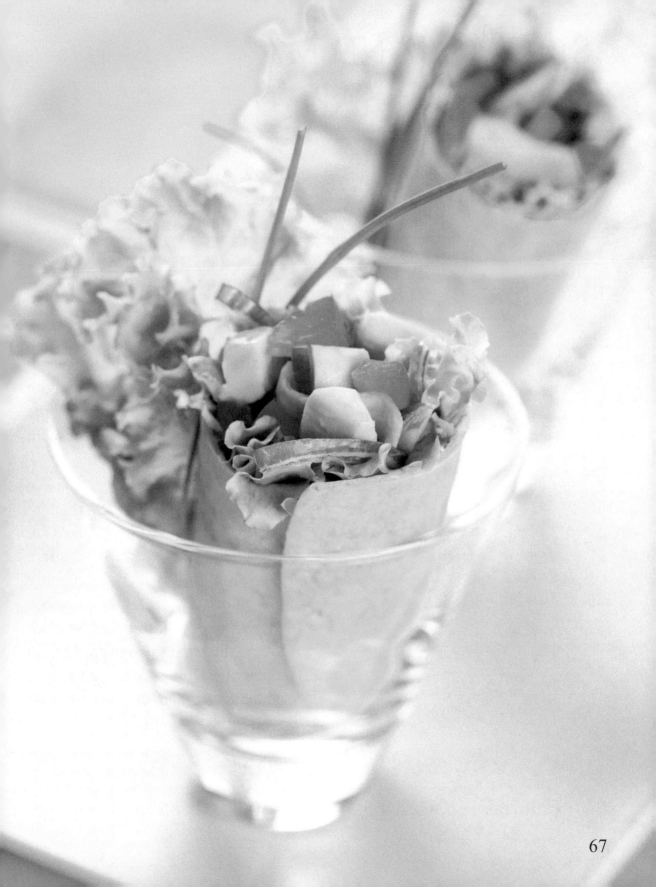

SPINACH AND MASHED TOFU SALAD

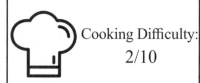 Cooking Difficulty: 2/10

 Cooking Time: 8 minutes

 Servings: 4

INGREDIENTS

- 16 oz. blocks firm tofu, drained
- 4 c. baby spinach leaves
- 4 tbsps. cashew butter
- 1½ tbsps. soy sauce
- 1-inch piece ginger, chopped
- 1 tsp. red miso paste
- 2 tbsps. sesame seeds
- 1 tsp. organic orange zest
- 1 tsp. nori flakes
- 2 tbsps. water

DESCRIPTION

STEP 1
Dry excess water left in the tofu using a paper towel before crumbling both blocks into small pieces. In a large bowl, combine the mashed tofu with the spinach leaves.

STEP 2
Mix the remaining ingredients in another small bowl and, if desired, add the optional water for a more smooth dressing. Pour this dressing over the mashed tofu and spinach leaves. Allow the salad to chill for up to one hour. Doing so will guarantee a better flavor. Or, the salad can be served right away. Enjoy!

NUTRITIONAL INFORMATION

Calories 166, Carbs 5.5 g, Fats 10.7 g, Protein 11.3 g

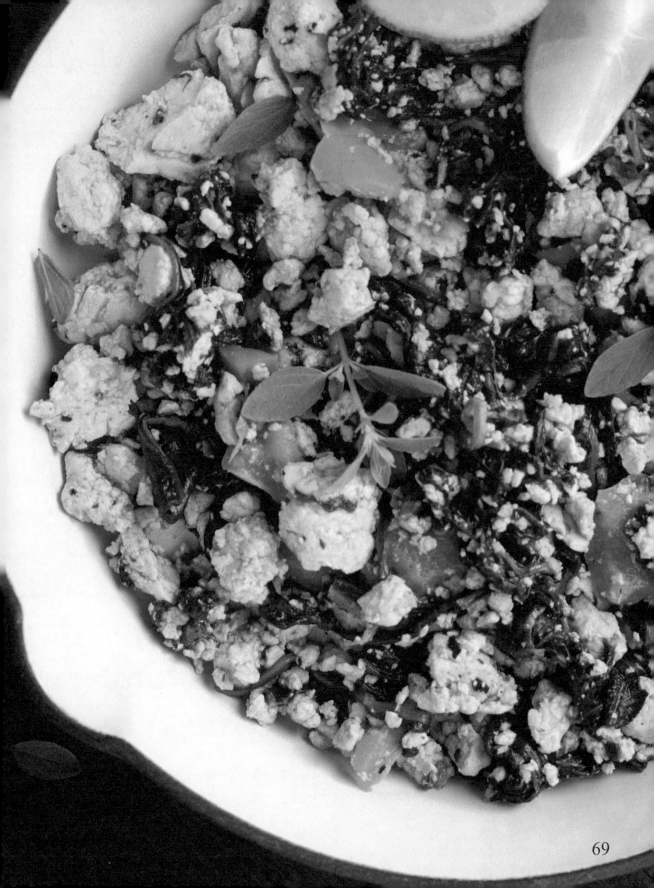

CUCUMBER EDAMAME SALAD

 Cooking Difficulty: 2/10

 Cooking Time: 15 minutes

 Servings: 2

INGREDIENTS

- 3 tbsps. avocado oil
- 1 c. cucumber, sliced
- ½ c. fresh sugar snap peas, sliced
- ½ c. fresh edamame
- ¼ c. radish, sliced
- 1 pitted hass avocado, peeled, sliced
- 1 crumbled nori sheet
- 2 tsps. roasted sesame seeds
- 1 tsp. salt

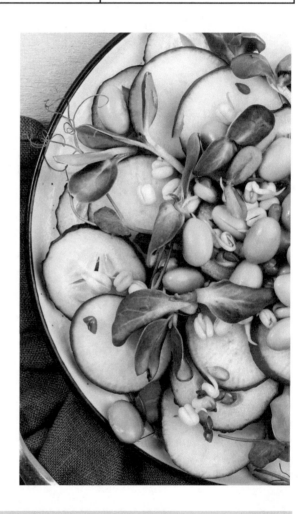

NUTRITIONAL INFORMATION

Calories 409, Carbs 7.1 g, Fats 38.25 g, Protein 7.6 g

DESCRIPTION

STEP 1
Bring a medium-sized pot filled halfway with water to a boil over medium-high heat.

STEP 2
Add the sugar snaps peas and cook them for about 2 minutes.

STEP 3
Take the pot off the heat, drain the excess water, transfer the sugar snaps peas to a medium-sized bowl and set aside for now.

STEP 4
Fill the pot with water again, add the teaspoon of salt and bring to a boil over medium-high heat.

STEP 5
Add in edamame and let them cook for about 6 minutes.

STEP 6
Take the pot off the heat, drain the excess water, transfer the soybeans to the bowl with sugar snaps peas, and let them cool down for about 5 minutes.

STEP 7
Using a bowl, mix all ingredients, except sesame seeds and nori crumbs.

STEP 8
Stir well to coat. Top with sesame seeds and nori crumbs.

STEP 9
Refrigerate for 30 minutes. Serve.

GARLIC CALAMARI MIX

 Cooking Difficulty: 2/10

 Cooking Time: 25 minutes

 Servings: 4

INGREDIENTS

- 3 minced garlic cloves
- 2 tbsps. olive oil
- 1 lb. calamari rings
- 1 tbsps. balsamic vinegar
- 1 c. vegetable stock
- salt
- black pepper
- ¼ c. chopped parsley

DESCRIPTION

STEP 1

Ensure that you heat the pan, add the garlic, stir, then cook for 5 minutes. Add the calamari and the other ingredients toss bring to a simmer then cook over medium heat for 20 minutes. Divide the mix into bowls and serve.

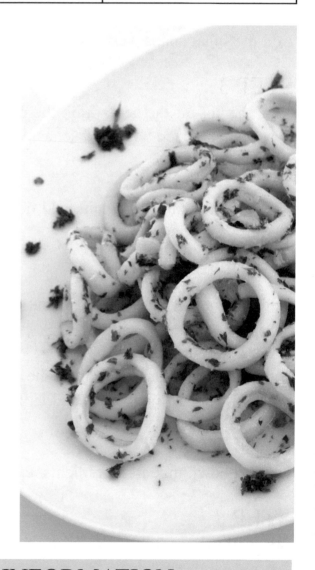

NUTRITIONAL INFORMATION

Calories 240, Fat 12g, Carbs 5.6g, Protein 25g

CHILI COD

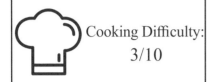 Cooking Difficulty: 3/10

 Cooking Time: 8 minutes

 Servings: 4

INGREDIENTS

- 4 boneless cod fillets
- 2 tbsps. avocado oil
- salt
- black pepper
- 1 tsp. chili powder
- 1 tbsp. chopped cilantro
- 3 minced garlic cloves
- ½ tsp. crushed chili pepper

DESCRIPTION

STEP 1

Heat up a pan with the oil over medium-high heat, add the garlic, chili pepper, and chili powder, stir then cook for 2 minutes. Add the fish and the other ingredients, cook for 5 minutes on each side, divide between plates and serve.

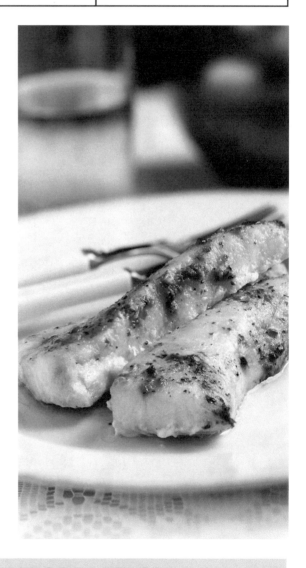

NUTRITIONAL INFORMATION

Calories 154, Fat 3g, Carbs 4g, Protein 24g

FIVE SPICE CHICKEN BREAST

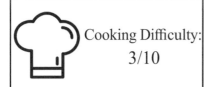 Cooking Difficulty: 3/10

 Cooking Time: 26 minutes

 Servings: 4

INGREDIENTS

- black pepper
- 1 tsp. five spice
- 1 tbsps. hot pepper
- 1 tbsp. avocado oil
- 1 tbsp. cilantro, chopped
- 2 chicken breast halves, skinless, deboned, and halved
- 1 c. tomatoes, crushed
- 2 tbsps. coconut aminos

DESCRIPTION

STEP 1
Heat up a pan with the oil over medium heat, add the meat and brown it for 2 minutes on each side.

STEP 2
Add the tomatoes, five spice, and the other ingredients, bring to a simmer, and cook over medium heat for 30 minutes.

STEP 3
Divide the whole mix between plates and serve.

NUTRITIONAL INFORMATION

Calories 244, Fat 8.4g, Carbs 4.5g, Protein 31g

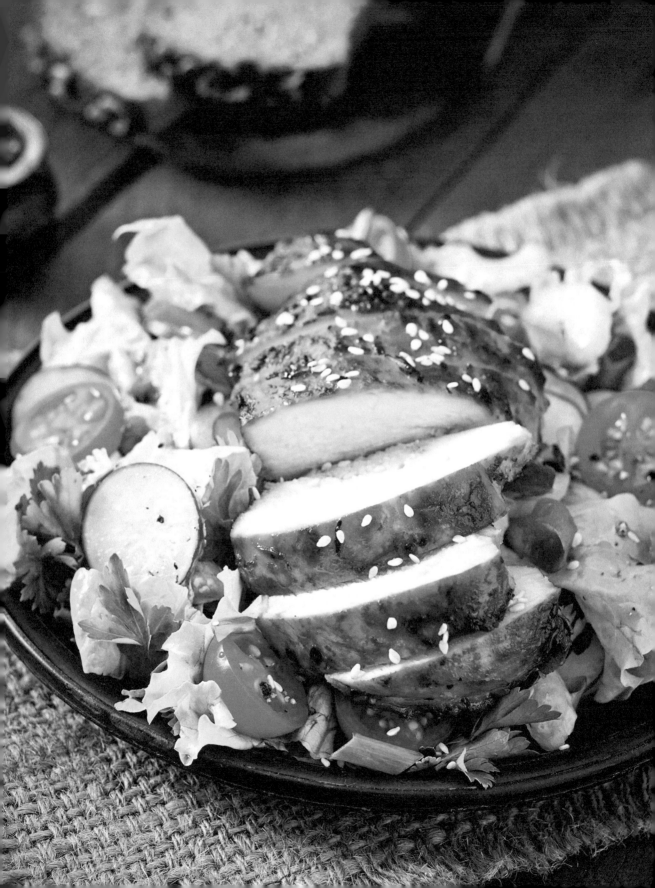

QUINOA EDAMAME SALAD

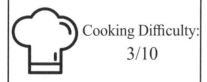 Cooking Difficulty: 3/10

 Cooking Time: 25 minutes

 Servings: 4

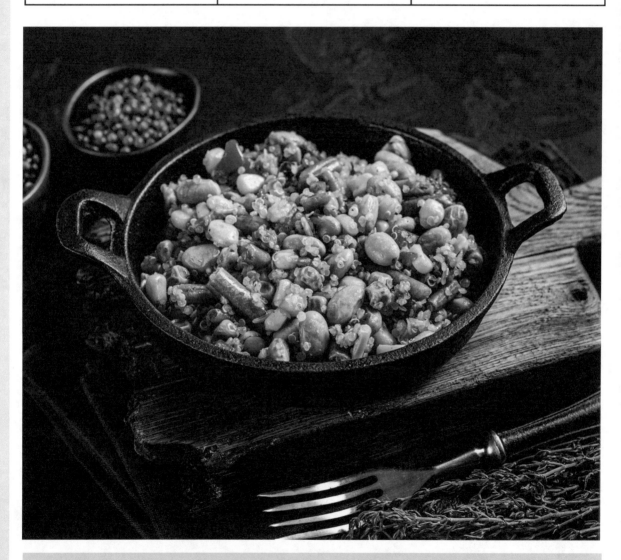

NUTRITIONAL INFORMATION

Calories: 295, Proteins: 7.6g, Carbs: 18.7g, Fat: 22.9g

INGREDIENTS

- 1 c. corn, frozen
- 1/8 tsp. black pepper, grounded
- 2 c. edamame shelled & frozen
- ¼ tsp. chilli powder
- 1 c. quinoa, cooked & cooled
- 1 tbsp. lime juice, fresh
- 1 green onion, sliced
- ¼ tsp. thyme, dried
- 2 tbsps. cilantro, fresh & chopped
- ¼ tsp. salt
- ½ red bell pepper, chopped
- 1 tbsp. lemon juice
- pinch of cayenne pepper
- 1 ½ tbsps. olive oil

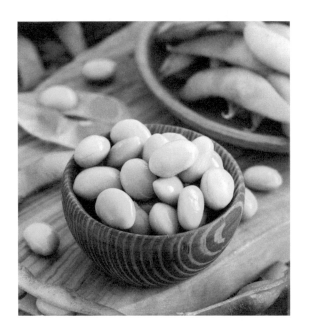

DESCRIPTION

STEP 1

Heat water in a large pot over medium heat. To this, stir in the edamame and corn.

STEP 2

Boil them slightly and cook them until they are tender.

STEP 3

Once cooked, drain the water and set it aside.

STEP 4

Now, combine all the remaining veggies and quinoa in a large bowl along with the cooked corn and edamame. Toss well.

STEP 5

In the meantime, to make the dressing, mix olive oil, lemon juice, lime juice, black pepper, thyme, chilli powder, and cayenne until emulsified.

STEP 6

Next, drizzle the dressing over the salad and place it in the refrigerator for at least 2 hours. Serve and enjoy.

APPLE LENTIL SALAD

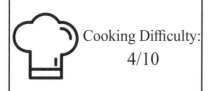 Cooking Difficulty: 4/10

 Cooking Time: 30 minutes

 Servings: 4

INGREDIENTS

- 2 c. lentil, dried
- ½ c. pepitas, roasted
- 1 tsp. salt
- 2 celery stalks, chopped
- 2 apples, chopped
- ¼ c. cranberries, dried
- 1 tbsp. rosemary, fresh & chopped
- 1 tbsp. lemon juice
- 2 tbsps. parsley, chopped
- dressing of your choice

DESCRIPTION

STEP 1

To start with, cook the lentils by following the instructions given in the packet until they are tender. Once cooked, allow them to cool and place them in the refrigerator until used.

STEP 2

Next, mix the apples with lemon juice in a bowl. Keep it in the refrigerator. After that, combine the chopped apples with the lentils and the remaining ingredients in the bowl.

STEP 3

Now, drizzle the dressing of your choice and place it in the refrigerator for at least an hour before serving. Serve and enjoy.

NUTRITIONAL INFORMATION

Calories: 431, Proteins: 26.5g, Carbs: 75.2g, Fat: 3.3g

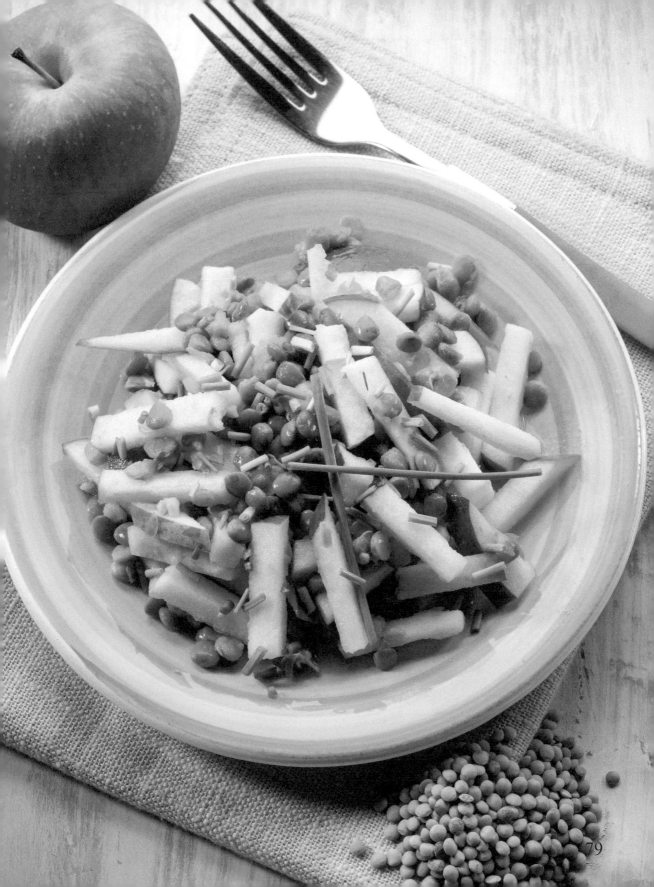

SWEET POTATO AND WHITE BEAN SKILLET

Cooking Difficulty: 4/10	Cooking Time: 30 minutes	Servings: 4

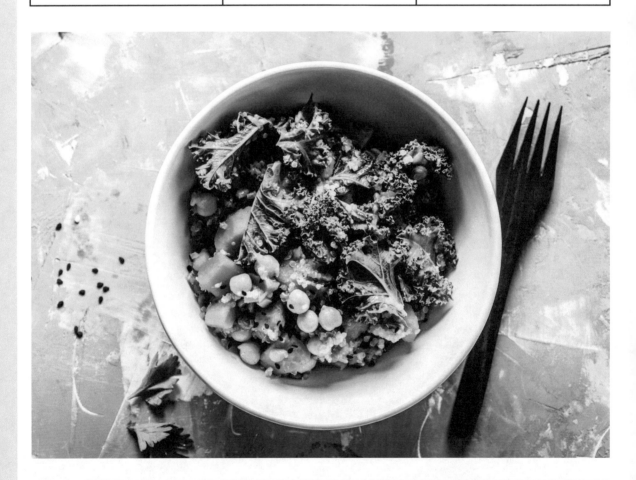

NUTRITIONAL INFORMATION

Calories: 263, Fat: 4 g, Carbs: 44 g, Protein: 13 g

INGREDIENTS

- 1 bunch kale, chopped
- 2 sweet potatoes, peeled, cubed
- 12 oz. cannellini beans
- 1 peeled onion, diced
- 1/8 tsp. red pepper flakes
- 1 tsp. salt
- 1 tsp. cumin
- ½ tsp. ground black pepper
- 1 tsp. curry powder
- 1 ½ tbsps. coconut oil
- 6 oz. coconut milk, unsweetened
- chickpeas (optional)

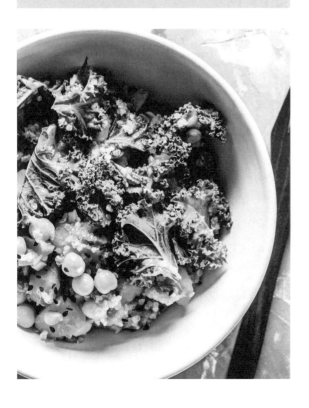

DESCRIPTION

STEP 1
Take a large skillet pan, place it over medium heat, add ½ tablespoon oil and when it melts, add onion and cook for 5 minutes.

STEP 2
Then stir in sweet potatoes, stir well, cook for 5 minutes, then season with all the spices, cook for 1 minute and remove the pan from heat.

STEP 3
Take another pan, add remaining oil in it, place it over medium heat and when oil melts, add kale, season with some salt and black pepper, stir well, pour in the milk and cook for 15 minutes until tender.

STEP 4
Then add beans, beans, and red pepper, stir until mixed and cook for 5 minutes until hot.

STEP 5
Serve straight away.

GREEN BEANS AND POTATOES

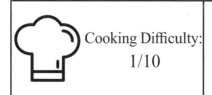 Cooking Difficulty:
1/10

 Cooking Time:
19 minutes

 Servings:
4

INGREDIENTS

- 1 pound green beans, trimmed
- 1 pound baby potatoes, halved
- 2 tablespoons olive oil
- 1 teaspoon garlic powder
- 1 teaspoon dried thyme
- 1/2 teaspoon salt
- 1/4 teaspoon black pepper
- cooking spray

DESCRIPTION

STEP 1
Preheat the air fryer to 375°F for 5 minutes. In a mixing bowl, toss the green beans and potatoes with olive oil, garlic powder, thyme, salt, and black pepper until evenly coated.

STEP 2
Spray the air fryer basket with cooking spray. Add the green beans and potatoes to the air fryer basket in a single layer.

STEP 3
Cook for 12-15 minutes, shaking the basket every 5 minutes until the green beans and potatoes are tender and lightly browned. Serve.

NUTRITIONAL INFORMATION

Calories 212, Fat 5g, Carbs 34g, Protein 5g

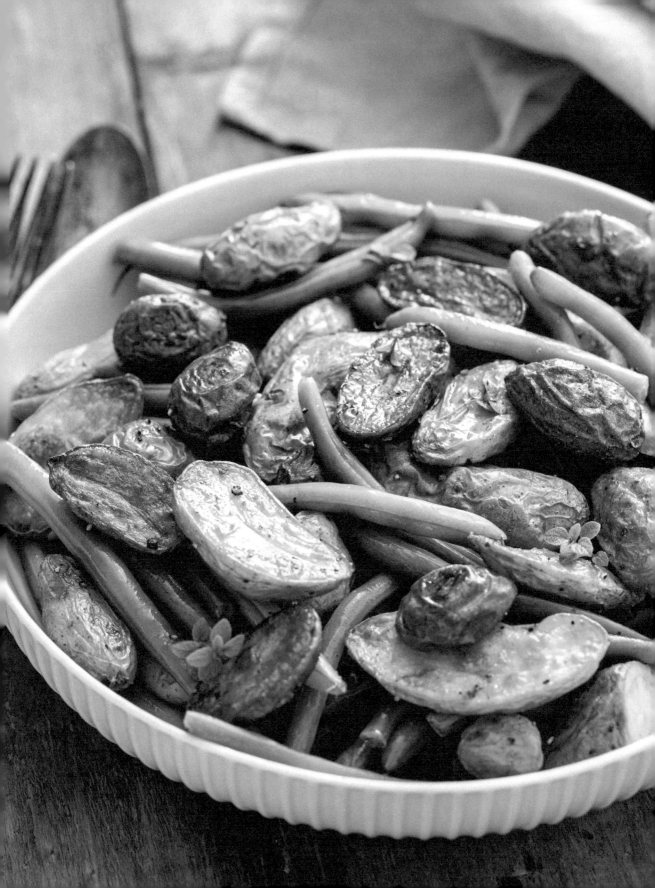

CHICKPEA AND SPINACH CUTLETS

 Cooking Difficulty: 3/10

 Cooking Time: 40 minutes

 Servings: 12

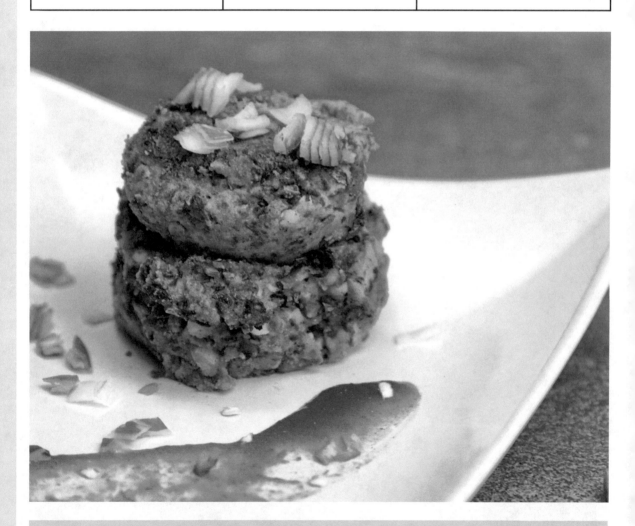

NUTRITIONAL INFORMATION

Calories: 200, Protein: 8 g, Fat: 11g, Carbs: 21 g

INGREDIENTS

- 1 red bell pepper
- 19 oz. chickpeas, rinsed & drained
- 1 c. ground almonds
- 2 tsps. dijon mustard
- 1 tsp. oregano
- ½ tsp. sage
- 1 c. spinach, fresh
- 1½ c. rolled oats
- 1 clove garlic, pressed
- ½ lemon, juiced
- 2 tsps. maple syrup, pure

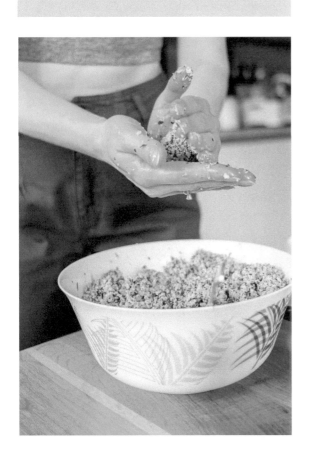

DESCRIPTION

STEP 1
Get out a baking sheet. Line it with parchment paper. Cut your red pepper in half and then take the seeds out. Place it on your baking sheet, and roast in the oven while you prepare your other ingredients.

STEP 2
Process your chickpeas, almonds, mustard, and maple syrup together in a food processor.

STEP 3
Add in your lemon juice, oregano, sage, garlic, and spinach, processing again. Make sure it's combined, but don't puree it.

STEP 4
Once your red bell pepper is softened, which should roughly take ten minutes, add this to the processor as well. Add in your oats, mixing well.

STEP 5
Form twelve patties, cooking in the oven for a half hour. They should be browned.

CHILI COLLARD GREENS

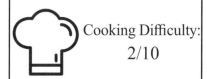 Cooking Difficulty: 2/10

 Cooking Time: 20 minutes

 Servings: 2

INGREDIENTS

- 1 tbsp. chili powder
- 1 bunch collard greens, chopped
- 1 tbsp. olive oil
- ½ c. vegetable stock
- 2 chopped shallots
- 1 tsp. hot paprika
- ½ tsp. cumin, ground
- salt
- black pepper
- 1 tbsp. lime juice

DESCRIPTION

STEP 1
Heat up a pan with the oil over medium-high heat; add the shallots and sauté for 5 minutes.

STEP 2
Add the collard greens and the other ingredients, toss, then cook over medium heat for 15 minutes more.

STEP 3
Divide everything between plates and serve.

NUTRITIONAL INFORMATION

Calories 245, Fat 20g, Carbs 5g, Protein 12g

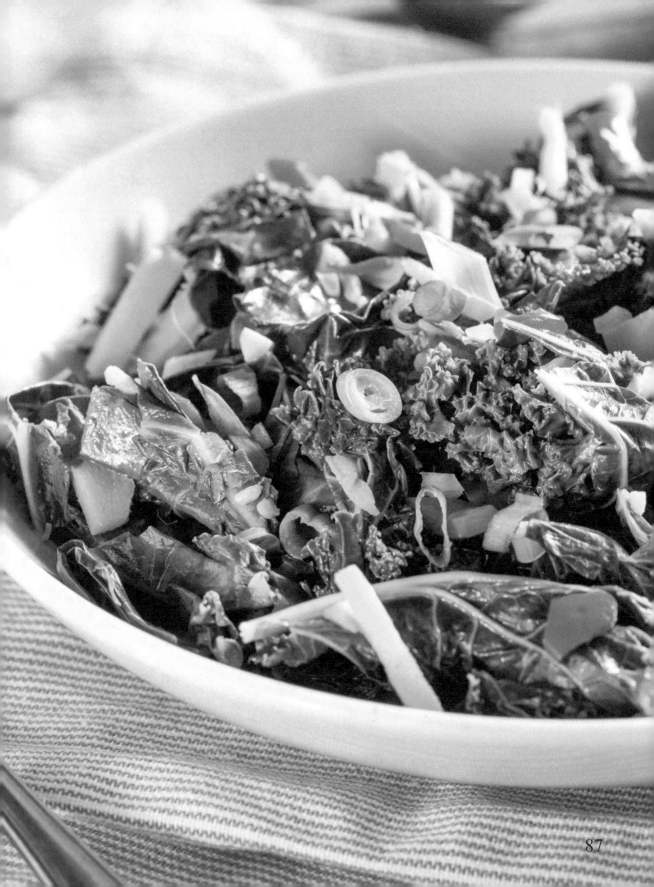

COCONUT CHICKPEA CURRY

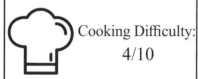 Cooking Difficulty: 4/10

 Cooking Time: 27 minutes

 Servings: 4

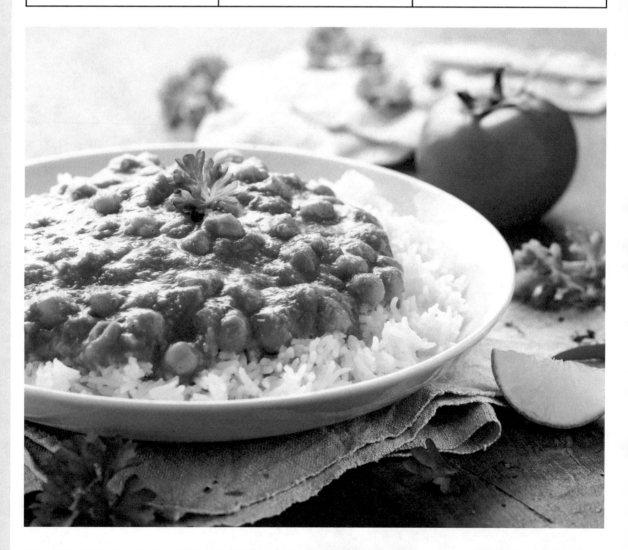

NUTRITIONAL INFORMATION

Calories: 225, Fat: 9.4 g, Carbs: 28.5 g, Protein: 7.3

INGREDIENTS

- 2 tsps. coconut flour
- 16 oz. cooked chickpeas
- 14 oz. tomatoes, diced
- 1 red onion, sliced
- 1 ½ tsps. minced garlic
- ½ tsp. sea salt
- 1 tsp. curry powder
- 1/3 tsp. ground black pepper
- 1 ½ tbsps. garam masala
- ¼ tsp. cumin
- 1 lime, juiced
- 13.5 oz. coconut milk, unsweetened
- 2 tbsps. coconut oil

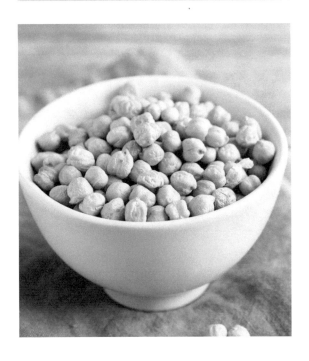

DESCRIPTION

STEP 1

Take a large pot, place it over medium-high heat, add oil and when it melts, add onions and tomatoes, season with salt and black pepper and cook for 5 minutes.

STEP 2

Switch heat to medium-low level, cook for 10 minutes until tomatoes have released their liquid, then add chickpeas and stir in garlic, curry powder, garam masala, and cumin until combined.

STEP 3

Stir in milk and flour, bring the mixture to boil, then switch heat to medium heat and simmer the curry for 12 minutes until cooked.

STEP 4

Taste to adjust seasoning, drizzle with lime juice, and serve. Place remaining portions in an airtight container and refrigerate for up to 2 days. Reheat before serving.

BALSAMIC-GLAZED ROASTED CAULIFLOWER

 Cooking Difficulty: 3/10

 Cooking Time: 75 minutes

 Servings: 4

INGREDIENTS

- 1 head cauliflower
- ½ lb. green beans, trimmed
- 1 peeled red onion, wedged
- 2 c. cherry tomatoes
- ½ tsp. salt
- ¼ c. brown sugar (optinal)
- 3 tbsps. olive oil
- 1 c. balsamic vinegar
- 2 tbsps. chopped parsley, for garnish

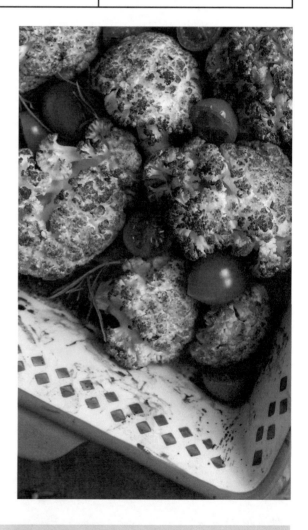

NUTRITIONAL INFORMATION

Calories: 225, Fat: 9.4 g, Carbs: 28.5 g, Protein: 7.3

STEP 1

Place cauliflower florets in a baking dish, add tomatoes, green beans, and onion wedges around it, season with salt, and drizzle with oil.

STEP 2

Pour vinegar in a saucepan, stir in sugar, bring the mixture to a boil and simmer for 15 minutes until reduced by half.

STEP 3

Brush the sauce generously over cauliflower florets and then roast for 1 hour at 400 degrees f until cooked, brushing sauce frequently.

STEP 4

When done, garnish vegetables with parsley and then serve.

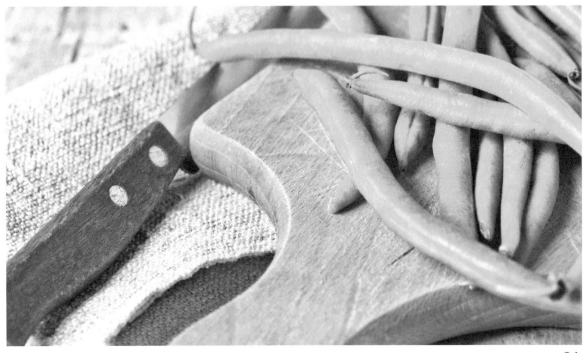

GARLICKY KALE & PEA SAUTÉ

 Cooking Difficulty: 2/10

 Cooking Time: 8 minutes

 Servings: 2

INGREDIENTS

- 2 sliced garlic cloves
- 1 chopped hot red chile
- 2 tbsps. olive oil
- 2 bunches chopped kale
- 1 lb. frozen peas

DESCRIPTION

STEP 1

In a saucepot, mix the ingredients except peas. Cook until the kale becomes tender for about 6 minutes. Add peas and cook for 2 more minutes.

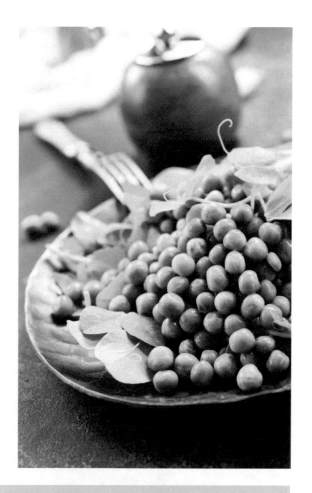

NUTRITIONAL INFORMATION

85 Calories, 3g Fats, 11g Net Carbs, and 5g Protein

SALAD WITH AVOCADO

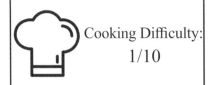 Cooking Difficulty: 1/10	Cooking Time: 6 minutes	Servings: 1

INGREDIENTS

- 1 avocado (diced)
- 1 tomato
- 1 cucumber (sliced)
- 1/4 red onion (thinly sliced)
- juice of half a lemon
- 1 tablespoon olive oil
- fresh herbs (cilantro, dill, or parsley)
- salt and pepper to taste

DESCRIPTION

STEP 1

Place all the diced vegetables in a bowl. Add lemon juice and olive oil. Gently toss all the ingredients until evenly coated. Season with salt and pepper to taste.

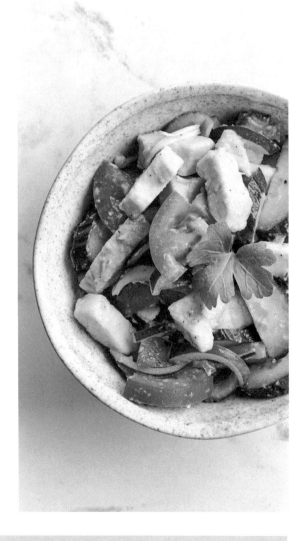

NUTRITIONAL INFORMATION

Calories 256, Fat 13.7g, Carbs 28.1g, Protein 6.7g

BLACK BEAN STUFFED SWEET POTATOES

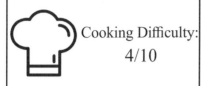 Cooking Difficulty: 4/10	Cooking Time: 80 minutes	Servings: 4

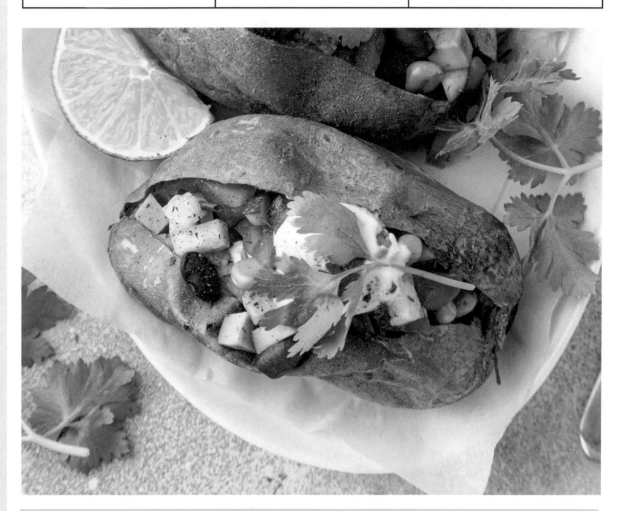

NUTRITIONAL INFORMATION

Calories: 387, Fat: 16.1 g, Carbs: 53 g, Protein: 10.4 g

INGREDIENTS

- 4 sweet potatoes
- 15 oz. cooked black beans
- ½ tsp. ground black pepper
- ½ red onion, peeled, diced
- ½ tsp. sea salt
- ¼ tsp. onion powder
- ¼ tsp. garlic powder
- ¼ tsp. red chili powder
- ¼ tsp. cumin
- 1 tsp. lime juice
- 1 ½ tbsps. olive oil
- ½ c. cashew cream sauce

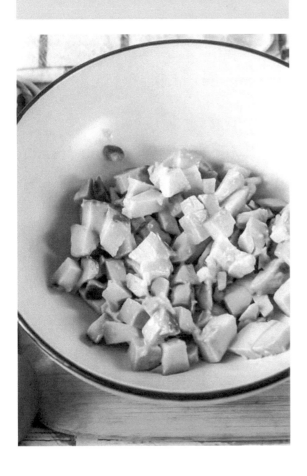

DESCRIPTION

STEP 1
Spread sweet potatoes on a baking tray greased with oil and bake for 65 minutes at 350 degrees f until tender.

STEP 2
Meanwhile, prepare the sauce, and for this, whisk together the cream sauce, black pepper, and lime juice until combined, set aside until required.

STEP 3
When 10 minutes of the baking time of potatoes are left, heat a skillet pan with oil. Add in onion to cook until golden for 5 minutes.

STEP 4
Then stir in spice, cook for another 3 minutes, stir in bean until combined and cook for 5 minutes until hot.

STEP 5
Let roasted sweet potatoes cool for 10 minutes, then cut them open, mash the flesh and top with bean mixture, cilantro and avocado, and then drizzle with cream sauce. Serve straight away.

SALMON AND POTATO SALAD

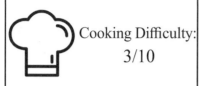 Cooking Difficulty: 3/10

 Cooking Time: 20 minutes

 Servings: 6

INGREDIENTS

- 1 tbsp. chopped parsley
- 6 oz. salmon
- 1 chopped onion
- 1 tbsp. olive oil
- 3 baking potatoes
- basil leaves

DESCRIPTION

STEP 1
Boil the potatoes until done. While those are boiling, heat up some oil in a pan and fry the onions.

STEP 2
Place the salmon slices into a dish and put the onions on top.

STEP 3
Top with the potatoes and sprinkle the parsley on top before serving and basil leaves.

NUTRITIONAL INFORMATION

120 Calories, 3.5g Fats, 20g Net Carbs, and 2g Protein

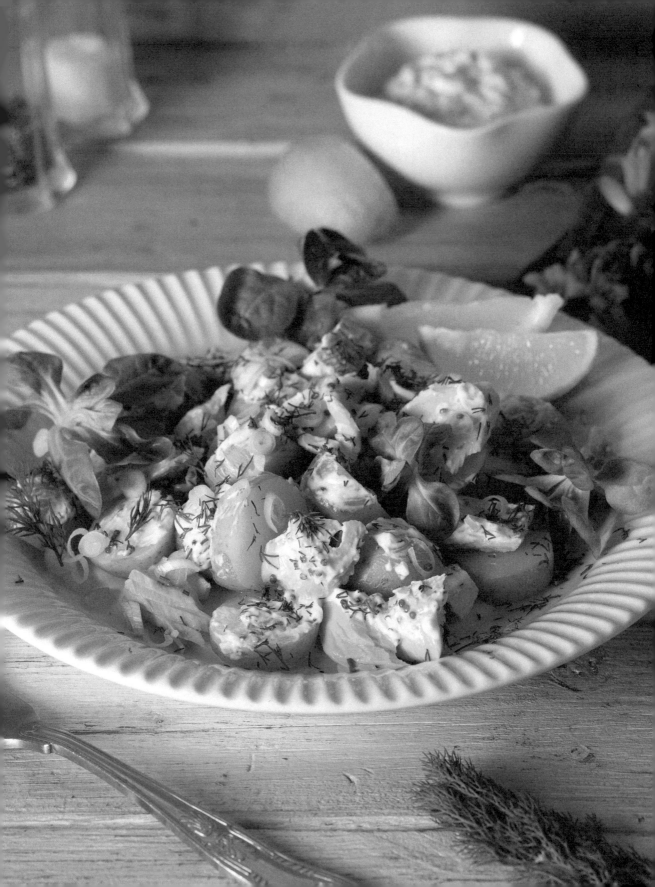

TASTY ROAST SALMON

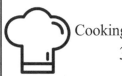 Cooking Difficulty: 3/10

 Cooking Time: 23 minutes

 Servings: 6

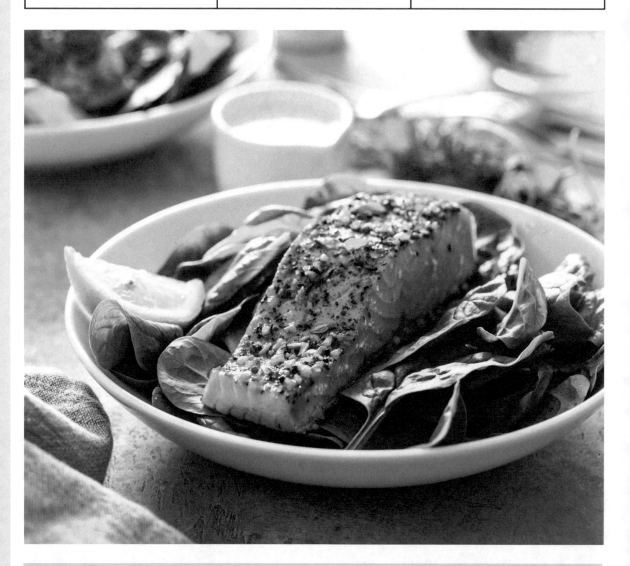

NUTRITIONAL INFORMATION

204.7 Calories, 10.4g Fats, 4.0g Net Carbs, 22.9g Protein

INGREDIENTS

- 1 medium size salmon
- 1 tbsp. olive oil
- 1 tbsp. white wine
- 1 tsp. paprika
- ½ tsp. ground ginger
- ½ tsp. crushed garlic
- 3 tsps. chopped parsley
- 1 lemon, cut into wedges

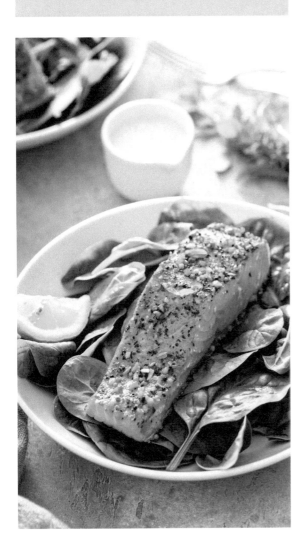

DESCRIPTION

STEP 1
Preheat oven to 400F.

STEP 2
Line a roasting tin with foil, or alternatively simply coat the tin with a little bit of olive oil.

STEP 3
In a good size bowl mix together the garlic, ginger, paprika, chopped parsley and season with salt and pepper. Stir the mix well and then add in the salmon, gently rubbing the marinade over the fish.

STEP 4
Lay the salmon in the prepared tin and top it with a dash of white wine. Roast the fish uncovered for about 20 minutes.

STEP 5
Put the cooked tasty salmon in your serving dish decorated with your choice of herbs and lemon. Make sure pour the remaining juice over the fish.

CORIANDER SHRIMP SALAD

 Cooking Difficulty: 2/10

 Cooking Time: 8 minutes

 Servings: 4

INGREDIENTS

- 1 tbsp. coriander, chopped
- 1 lb. shrimp, deveined and peeled
- 1 red onion, sliced
- ¼ tsp. black pepper
- 2 c. baby arugula
- 1 tbsp. lemon juice
- 1 tbsp. olive oil
- 1 tbsp. balsamic vinegar

DESCRIPTION

STEP 1
Heat up a pan with the oil over medium heat, add the onion, stir and sauté for 2 minutes.

STEP 2
Add the shrimp and the other ingredients, toss, cook for 6 minutes, divide into bowls and serve for lunch.

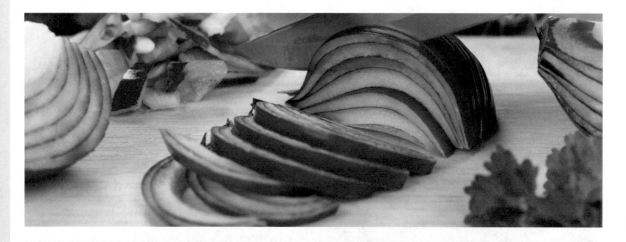

NUTRITIONAL INFORMATION

Calories 341, Fat 11.5g, Carbs 17.3g, Protein 14.3g

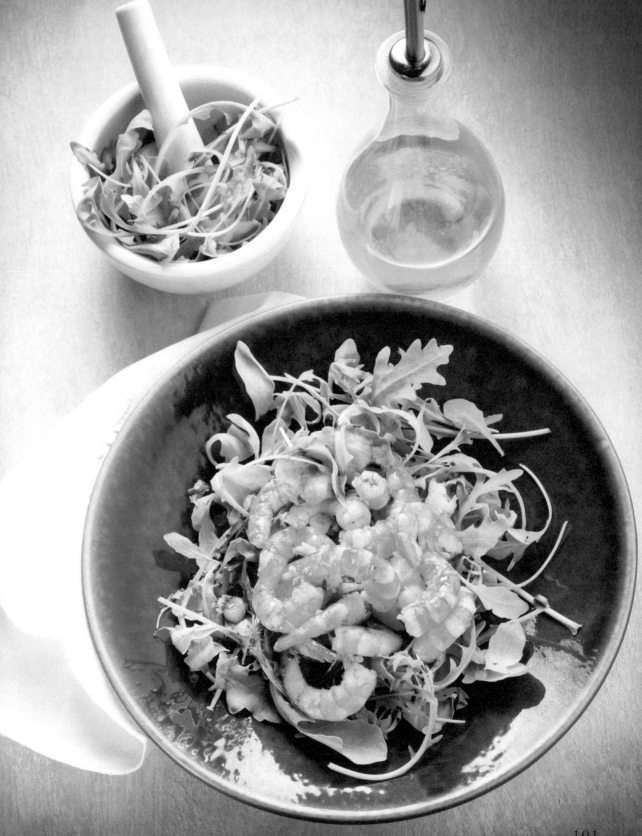

ROASTED COD WITH BOK CHOY

 Cooking Difficulty: 3/10

 Cooking Time: 20 minutes

 Servings: 4

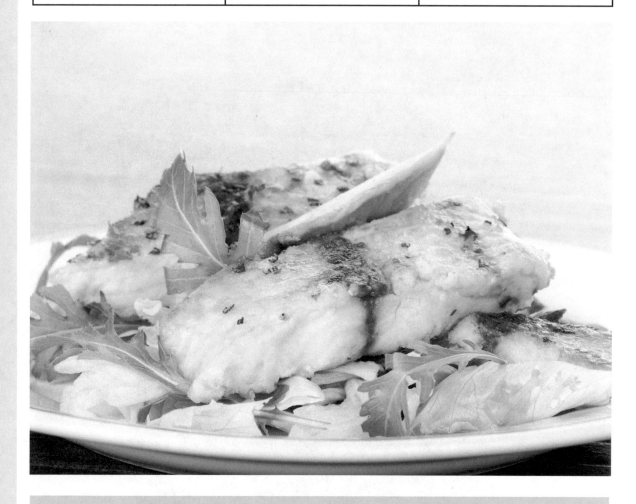

NUTRITIONAL INFORMATION

355 Calories, 21g Fats, 3g Net Carbs, and 37g Protein

INGREDIENTS

- 24 oz. cod fillets
- ¾ lb. baby bok choy
- olive oil
- 1 tbsps. granulated garlic
- salt
- black pepper

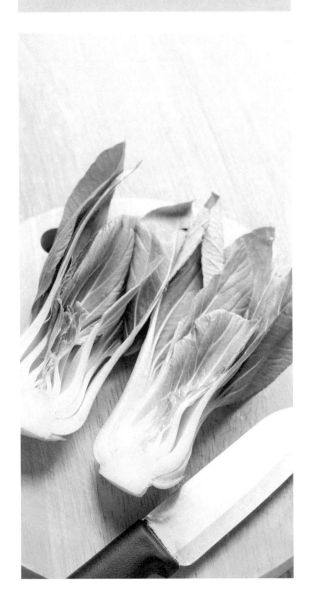

DESCRIPTION

STEP 1
Set the oven to 400 degrees F to preheat.

STEP 2
Cut out 3 sheets of aluminum foil, each large enough to completely cover one cod fillet.

STEP 3
Place a cod fillet on each sheet of aluminum foil then add the olive oil and granulated garlic. Add the bok choy, then season everything with salt and pepper.

STEP 4
Fold over the pouches and crimp the edges. Arrange on a baking sheet.

STEP 5
Bake for 20 minutes, then transfer to a cooling rack.

STEP 6
Let cool slightly, then refrigerate for up to 3 days. Reheat in the oven before serving.

SALMON CUTLETS

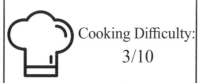 Cooking Difficulty: 3/10

 Cooking Time: 15 minutes

 Servings: 3

INGREDIENTS

- 6 oz. salmon
- 1 small sweet potato
- 1 egg
- 1 tsp. pepper
- 1 tsp. salt
- 2 tbsps. fresh dill
- 2 tbsp. melted coconut oil
- 2 sliced scallions

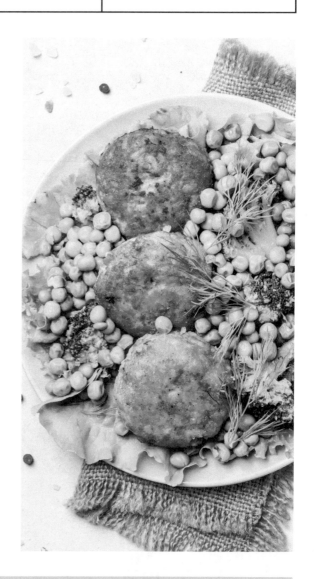

NUTRITIONAL INFORMATION

260 Calories, 8g Carbs, 28g Protein, 12g Fat

DESCRIPTION

STEP 1

Pre-heat your oven to 425 degrees Fahrenheit. Drain the canned salmon.

STEP 2

Microwave the sweet potato for 2 minutes or until tender and can be cut easily. Don't forget to poke holes in it before placing it in the microwave.

STEP 3

In a big bowl, combine the egg, pepper, salmon, scallions and dill.

STEP 4

Slice the sweet potato in half and remove the skin. Allow cooling. Add it into the salmon mix.

STEP 5

Use parchment paper to line a baking sheet, brush melted coconut oil on it.

STEP 6

Scoop 1/3 c. of salmon mixture and place it on the baking sheet. Flatten into half-inch thick, make sure that the thickness is even throughout.

STEP 7

Bake for 20 mins. then flip and cook until the patties start to brown for 10 minutes or cooked through.

STEP 8

Serve together with tartar sauce or with English muffins.

SHRIMP SALAD

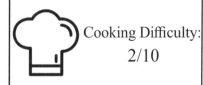 Cooking Difficulty: 2/10

 Cooking Time: 8 minutes

 Servings: 4

INGREDIENTS

- 1 lb. shrimp, deveined and peeled
- 1 red onion, sliced
- ¼ tsp. black pepper
- 2 c. baby arugula
- 1 tbsp. lemon juice
- 1 tbsp. olive oil

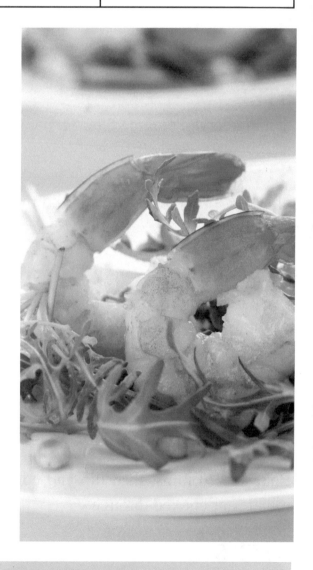

DESCRIPTION

STEP 1

Heat up a pan with the oil over medium heat, add the onion, stir and sauté for 2 minutes. Add the shrimp and the other ingredients, toss, cook for 6 minutes, divide into bowls and serve.

NUTRITIONAL INFORMATION

Calories 341, Fat 11.5g, Carbs 17.3g, Protein 14.3g

SALMON AND SHRIMP BOWLS

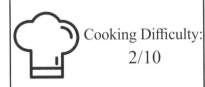 Cooking Difficulty: 2/10

 Cooking Time: 12 minutes

 Servings: 4

INGREDIENTS

- ½ c. mild salsa
- 1 tbsp. olive oil
- ½ lb. shrimp, peeled and deveined
- 1 red onion, chopped
- 2 tbsps. cilantro, chopped
- ½ lb. smoked salmon
- ¼ c. tomatoes, cubed

DESCRIPTION

STEP 1

Heat up a pan with the oil over medium-high heat, add the salmon, toss and cook for 5 minutes. Add the onion, shrimp, and the other ingredients, cook for 7 minutes more, divide into bowls, and serve.

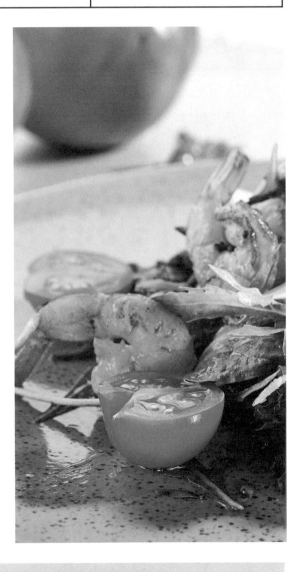

NUTRITIONAL INFORMATION

Calories 251, Fat 11.4g, Carbs 12.3g, Protein 7.1g

CHEESY TURKEY PAN

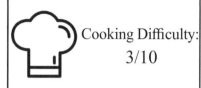 Cooking Difficulty: 3/10

 Cooking Time: 25 minutes

 Servings: 4

INGREDIENTS

- 2 c. grated cheddar cheese
- 1 boneless turkey breast, skinless and cubed
- 1 tbsp. tomato passata
- ¼ c. veggie stock
- 1 tbsp. olive oil
- 2 chopped shallots
- ¼ c. cubed tomatoes
- salt and black pepper
- pasta

DESCRIPTION

STEP 1
Ensure that you heat the pan; add the shallots and sauté for 2 minutes.

STEP 2
Add the meat and brown for 5 minutes.

STEP 3
Add the pasta and the other ingredients except for the cheese toss, then cook over medium heat for 10 minutes more.

STEP 4
Sprinkle the cheese on top, cook everything for 7-8 minutes, divide between plates, and serve.

NUTRITIONAL INFORMATION

Calories 309, Fat 23.1g, Carbs 3.9g, Protein 21.6g

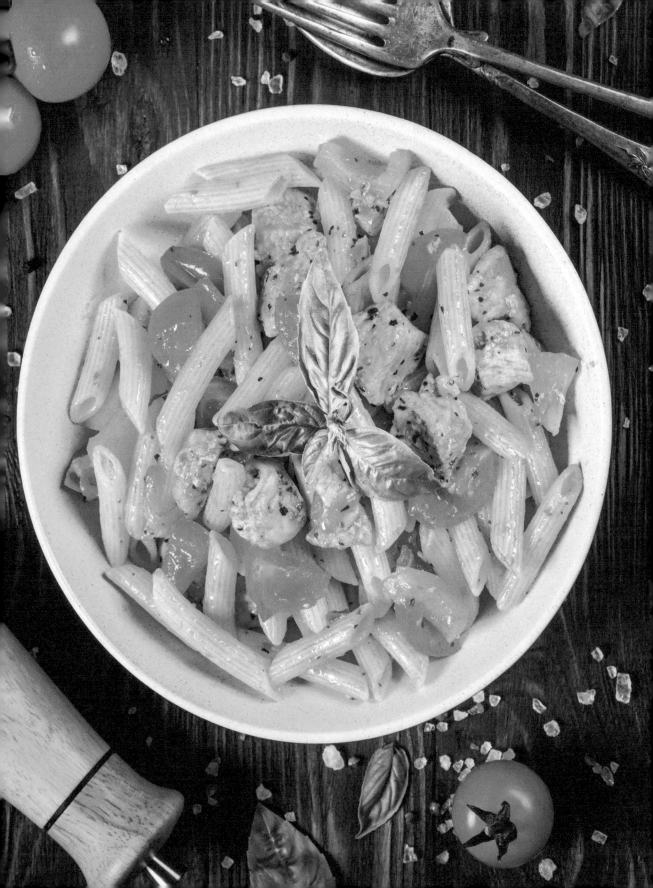

TURKEY AND ENDIVES SALAD

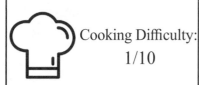 Cooking Difficulty: 1/10

 Cooking Time: 2 minutes

 Servings: 4

INGREDIENTS

- 1 sliced cooked turkey breast, skinless and boneless
- 2 tbsps. avocado oil
- 2 shredded endives
- 1 c. halved cherry tomatoes
- 2 tbsps. lime juice
- 2 tbsps. balsamic vinegar
- 2 tbsps. chopped chives
- black pepper

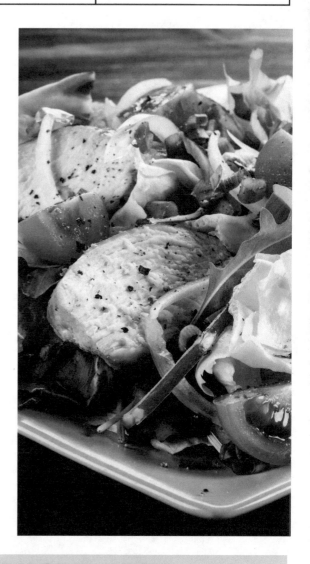

DESCRIPTION

STEP 1

In a bowl, mix the turkey with the endives and the other ingredients, toss and serve for lunch.

NUTRITIONAL INFORMATION

Calories 200, Fat 10g, Carbs 3g, Protein 7g

CHICKEN SALAD

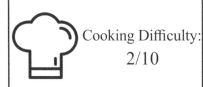 Cooking Difficulty: 2/10

 Cooking Time: 3 minutes

 Servings: 4

INGREDIENTS

- ¼ tsp. black pepper
- 1 red onion, chopped
- 2 rotisserie chicken, de-boned, skinless and shredded
- ¼ c. walnuts, chopped
- 1 lb. cherry tomatoes, halved
- green pea
- 2 tbsps. lemon juice
- 1 tbsp. olive oil
- 4 c. baby spinach

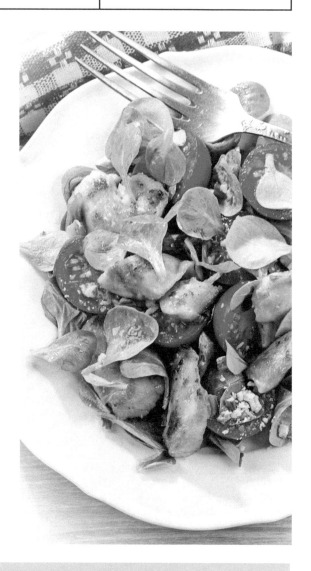

DESCRIPTION

STEP 1

In a salad bowl, combine the chicken with the tomato and the other ingredients, toss and serve.

NUTRITIONAL INFORMATION

Calories 380, Fat 40g, Carbs 1g, Protein 17g

CHICKEN PIECES

 Cooking Difficulty: 3/10

 Cooking Time: 15 minutes

 Servings: 6

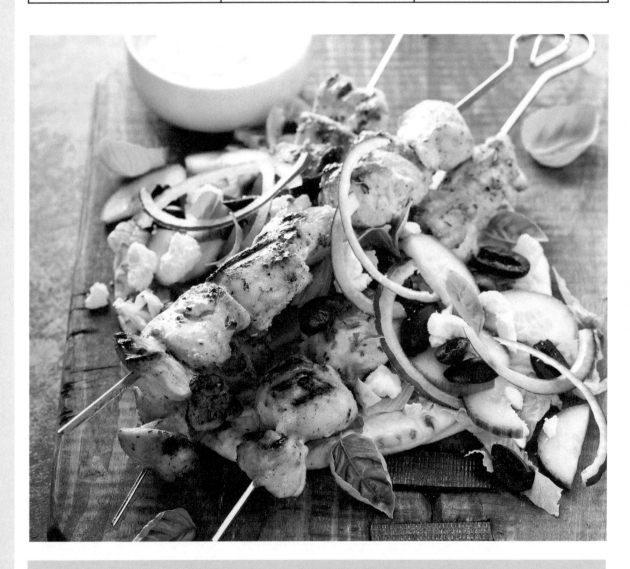

NUTRITIONAL INFORMATION

294 Calories, 5.2g Fat, 42.1g Carbs, 22.2g Protein

INGREDIENTS

- 2 tbsps. lime juice
- 14 oz. Greek yogurt
- 2 tsps. oregano
- ¼ c. white dry wine
- ¼ c. olive oil
- ½ tsp. pepper
- 1 tsp. kosher salt
- 2 lb. skinned breasts
- 1 tsp. granulated garlic
- 2 tsps. distilled white vinegar
- ½ c. cucumber

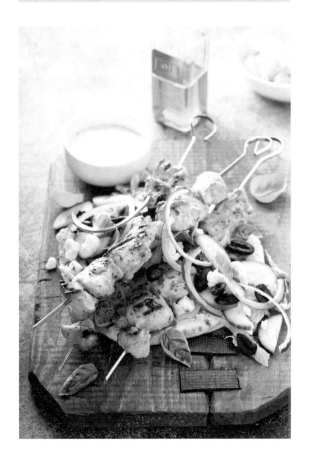

DESCRIPTION

STEP 1
Cut the chicken into ½-inch cubes, and coarsely shred the cucumber. Set the grill between 450°F and 550°F.

STEP 2
Blend the wine, oil, chicken, oregano, lime juice, ¼ teaspoon of the pepper, and the salt in a mixing bowl.

STEP 3
Use eight metal skewers to prepare the chicken for cooking. Grill for approximately 10-12 minutes.

STEP 4
Remove any excess moisture from the cucumbers with paper towels, and put them into a medium dish. Mix in the yogurt, garlic, vinegar, and pepper with the cucumbers.

STEP 5
Serve with warm pita bread and the chicken. Place remaining portions in an airtight container and refrigerate for up to 4 days. Reheat before serving.

BAKED CHICKEN WITH SWEET PAPRIKA

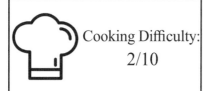 Cooking Difficulty: 2/10

 Cooking Time: 35 minutes

 Servings: 2

INGREDIENTS

- 2 chicken fillets
- 1 tbsp. sweet paprika
- 2 tbsp. olive oil
- 1 tbsp. dried garlic
- salt
- black pepper

DESCRIPTION

STEP 1
Preheat oven to 360 F.

STEP 2
Rub the chicken fillet with spices and olive oil and let sit for 5 minutes.

STEP 3
Place the chicken in the oven and bake for 30 minutes.

STEP 4
Serve with salad.

NUTRITIONAL INFORMATION

Calories 298, Fat 9,3g, Carbs 6g, Protein 11g

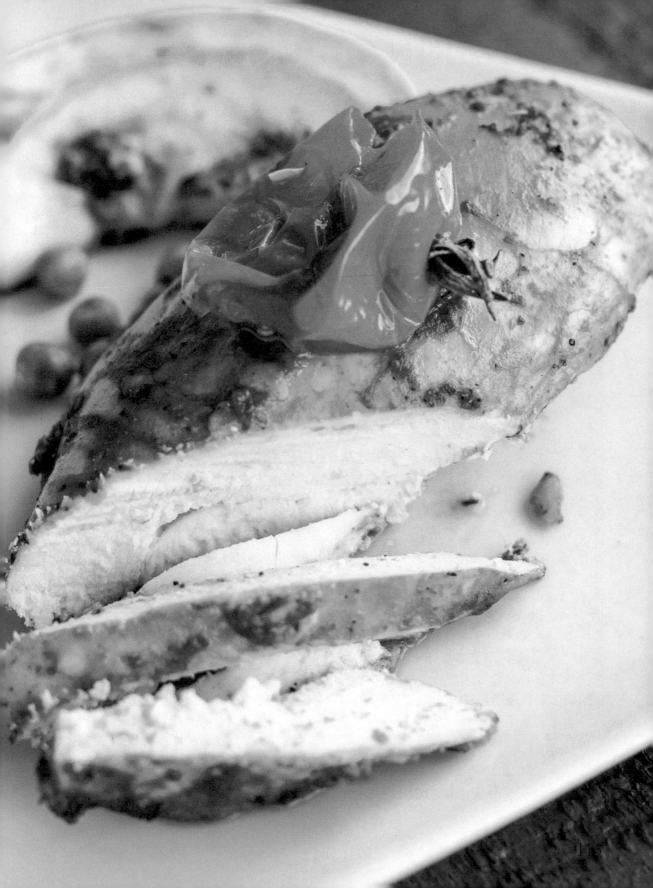

MANDARIN CHICKEN STIR FRY

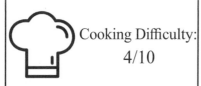 Cooking Difficulty: 4/10	Cooking Time: 25 minutes	Servings: 2

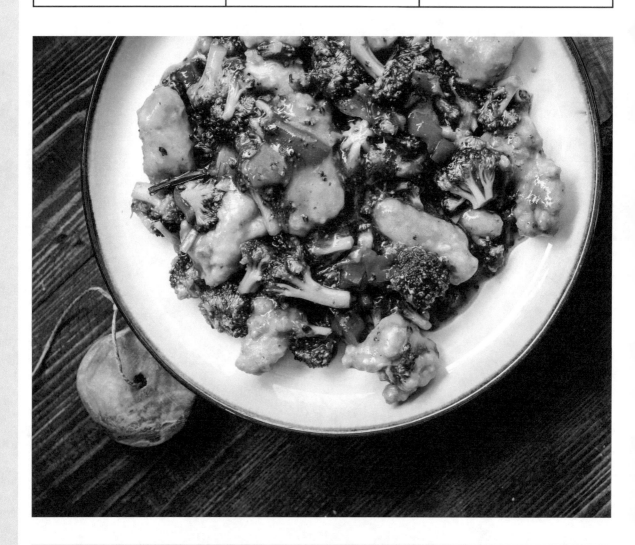

NUTRITIONAL INFORMATION

260 Calories, 8g Carbs, 28g Protein, 12g Fat

INGREDIENTS

- ½ c. broccoli, steamed
- 1 tsp. olive oil
- 1 boneless chicken breast, cubed
- ¾ c. freshly sliced mushroom
- juice of ½ orange
- 1 c. chicken stock
- 1 c. sliced fresh mandarin oranges, peeled
- 2 tbsps. green onion
- 1½ tsps. flour
- salt
- pepper
- ¼ c. onion

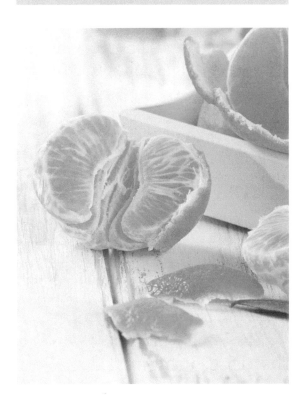

DESCRIPTION

STEP 1
Heat oil over high heat. Sauté the onion if using.

STEP 2
Stir in the chicken and cook until it's no longer pink.

STEP 3
Add mushroom and cook for three minutes.

STEP 4
In another pan, mix flour and orange juice. Add about 1/3 cup of water.

STEP 5
Bring to a boil and simmer until the sauce is thick enough.

STEP 6
Add the chicken and mushroom. Mix thoroughly.

STEP 7
Add the orange wedges and the broccoli. Season with salt and pepper.

STEP 8
Serve as it is or over rice or noodles.

SHRIMP AND ASPARAGUS SALAD

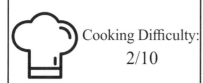 Cooking Difficulty: 2/10

 Cooking Time: 12 minutes

 Servings: 4

INGREDIENTS

- ¼ c. raspberry vinegar
- 2 tbsps. olive oil
- 2 c. cherry tomatoes halved (optional)
- 2 lbs. shrimp, peeled and deveined
- ¼ tsp. black pepper
- 1 lb. asparagus, pre-cooked
- 1 tbsps. lemon juice

DESCRIPTION

STEP 1
Heat up a pan with the oil over medium-high heat, add the shrimp, toss and cook for 2 minutes.

STEP 2
Add the asparagus and the other ingredients, toss, cook for 8 minutes more, divide into bowls, and serve.

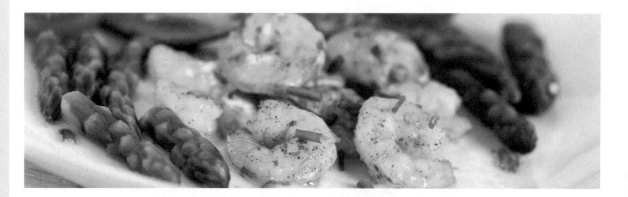

NUTRITIONAL INFORMATION

Calories: 79, Fat: 0.4 g, Carbs: 15 g, Protein: 1.3 g

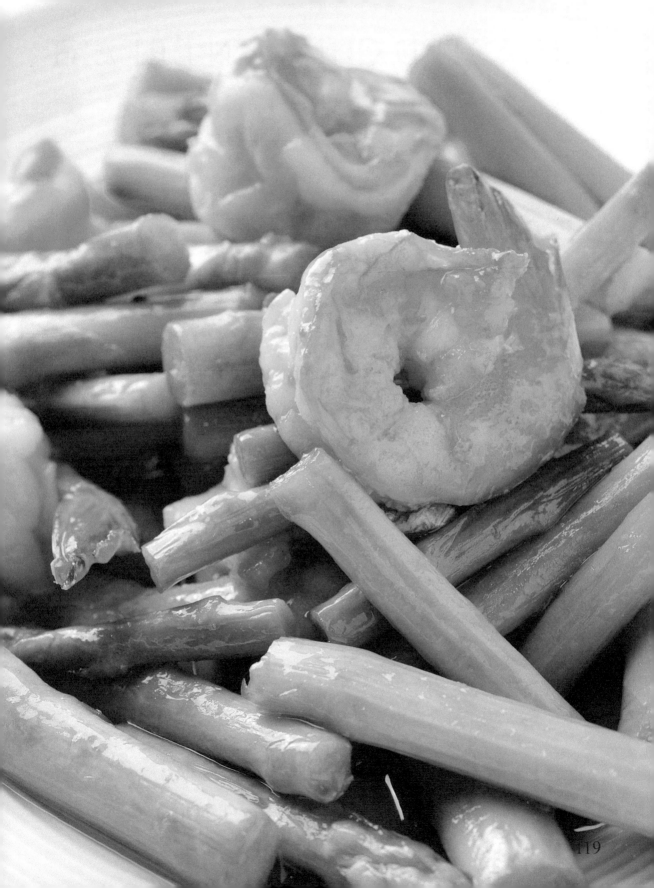

ROASTED CHICKEN BREAST AND VEGETABLES

 Cooking Difficulty: 4/10

 Cooking Time: 45 minutes

 Servings: 4

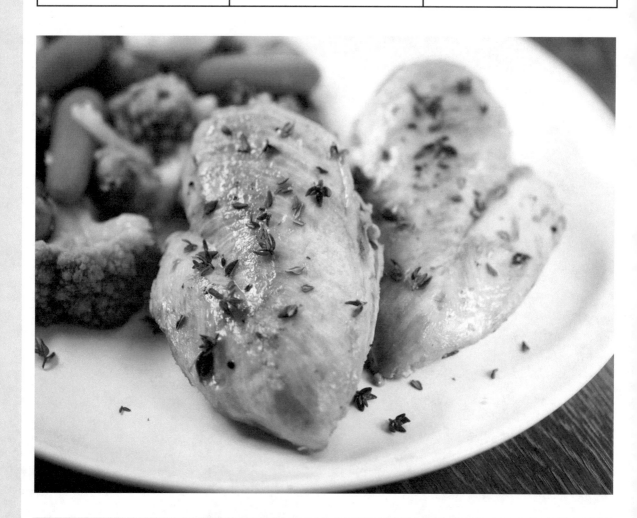

NUTRITIONAL INFORMATION

Calories: 276, Fat: 12.2g, Carbs: 17.4 g, Protein: 25.1g

INGREDIENTS

- 4 chicken breasts
- 1 tbsp. dijon mustard
- 1 tbsp. honey
- ½ tsp. garlic powder
- ½ tsp. dried rosemary
- ½ tsp. cayenne pepper
- 2 tbsps. olive oil
- 2 tbsps. lemon juice
- 1 tsp. minced garlic
- ½ tsp. dried basil
- 2 c. broccoli florets
- 2 sliced carrot
- 1 lb. marbled potatoes washed thoroughly
- salt and pepper

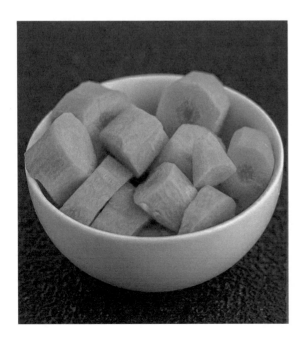

DESCRIPTION

STEP 1
Preheat your Air Fryer to 360°F.

STEP 2
In a shallow dish, place the chicken breast. Add the mustard, honey, garlic powder, rosemary, and cayenne pepper. Mix to coat well.

STEP 3
In a bowl, combine the olive oil, lemon juice, garlic, and basil. Add the vegetables and toss to coat. Season with salt and pepper.

STEP 4
Place the vegetables in the Air Fryer cooking basket and cook for 20-25 minutes, or until potatoes are tender. Transfer vegetables to a plate and tent with foil to keep warm.

STEP 5
Place the marinated chicken breasts inside the same Air Fryer cooking basket and cook for about 20 minutes or until cooked through. Serve chicken with roasted vegetables on the side. Enjoy!

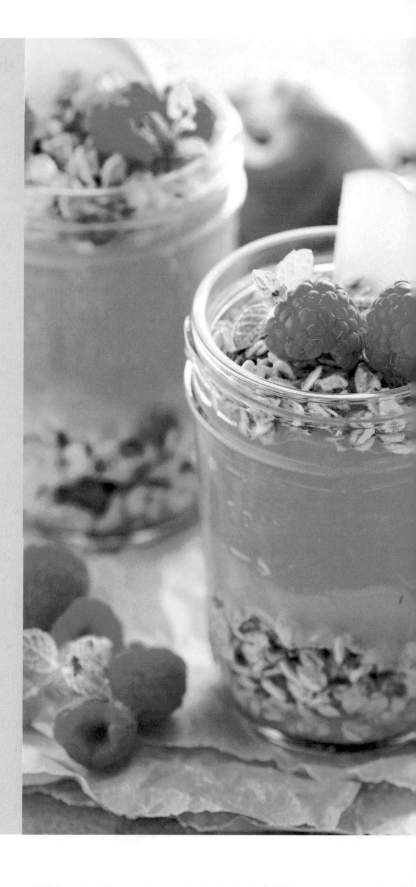

SNACKS & DESSERTS

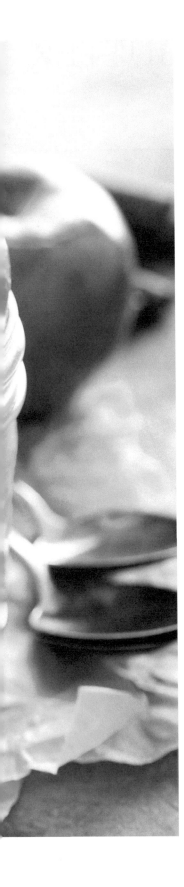
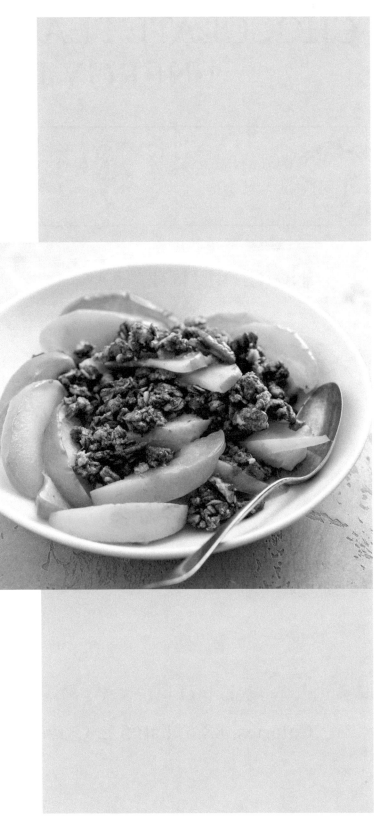

CHOCOLATE PEANUT BUTTER ENERGY BITES

 Cooking Difficulty: 1/10

 Cooking Time: 4 minutes

 Servings: 4

INGREDIENTS

- ½ c. oats, old-fashioned
- 1/3 c. cocoa powder, unsweetened
- 1 c. dates, chopped
- ½ c. shredded coconut flakes, unsweetened
- ½ c. peanut butter

DESCRIPTION

STEP 1
Place oats in a food processor along with dates and pulse for 1 minute until the paste starts to come together.

STEP 2
Then add remaining ingredients, and blend until incorporated and very thick mixture comes together.

STEP 3
Shape the mixture into balls, refrigerate for 1 hour until set and then serve.

NUTRITIONAL INFORMATION

Calories: 88.6, Fat: 5 g, Carbs: 10 g, Protein: 2.3 g

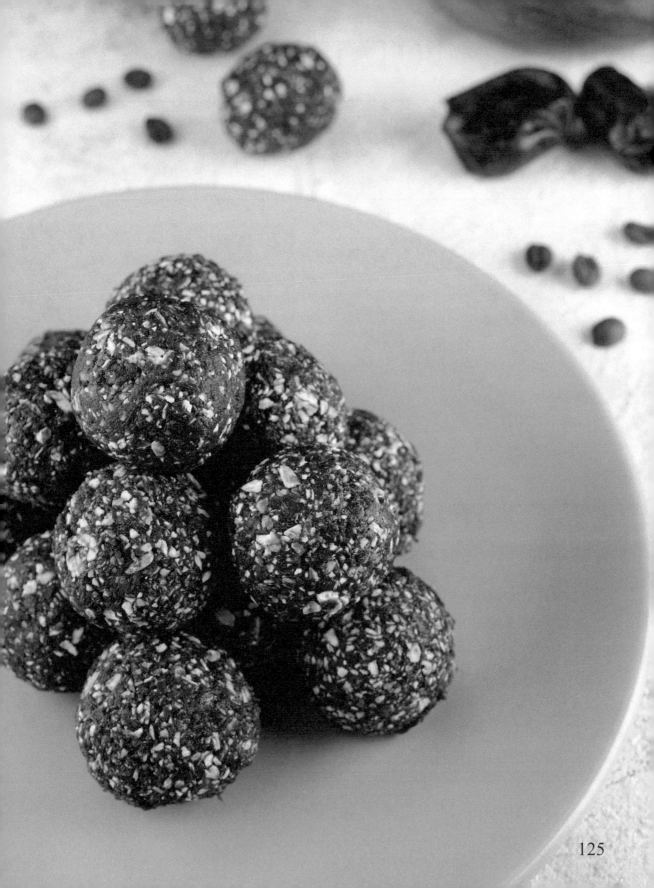

POTATO CHIPS

 Cooking Difficulty: 2/10

 Cooking Time: 21 minutes

 Servings: 4

INGREDIENTS

- 1 tsp. sweet paprika
- 1 tbsp. chives, chopped
- 4 gold potatoes, peeled and thinly sliced
- 2 tbsps. olive oil
- 1 tbsp. chili powder

DESCRIPTION

STEP 1

Spread the chips on a lined baking sheet, add the oil and the other ingredients, toss, introduce in the oven and bake at 390 degrees F for 20 minutes. Divide into bowls and serve.

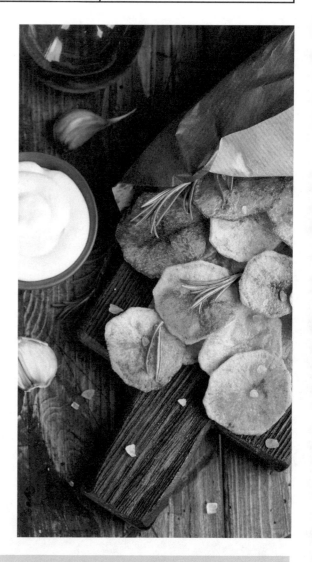

NUTRITIONAL INFORMATION

Calories 118, Fat 7.4g, Carbs 13.4g, Protein 1.3g

BEETS CHIPS

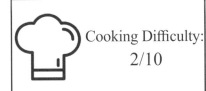 Cooking Difficulty: 2/10

 Cooking Time: 37 minutes

 Servings: 4

INGREDIENTS

- 1 tbsp. olive oil
- 2 tsps. garlic, minced
- 2 beets, peeled and thinly sliced
- 1 tsp. cumin, ground

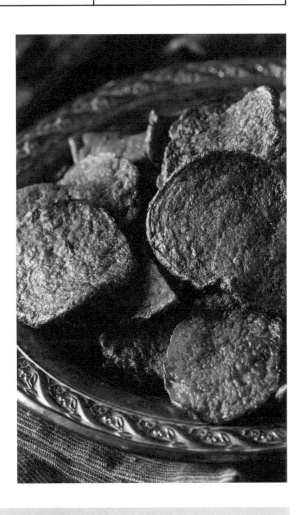

DESCRIPTION

STEP 1

Spread the beet chips on a lined baking sheet, add the oil and the other ingredients, toss, introduce in the oven and bake at 400 degrees F for 35 minutes. Divide into bowls and serve as a snack.

NUTRITIONAL INFORMATION

Calories 32, Fat 0.7g, Carbs 6.1g, Protein 1.1g

LENTILS SPREAD

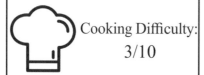 Cooking Difficulty: 3/10

 Cooking Time: 15 minutes

 Servings: 4

INGREDIENTS

- 2 garlic cloves, minced
- ½ c. cilantro, chopped
- 14 oz. canned lentils, drained, unsalted, and rinsed
- 1 lemon juice
- 2 tbsps. olive oil

DESCRIPTION

STEP 1

In a blender, combine the lentils with the oil and the other ingredients, pulse well, divide into bowls and serve as a party spread.

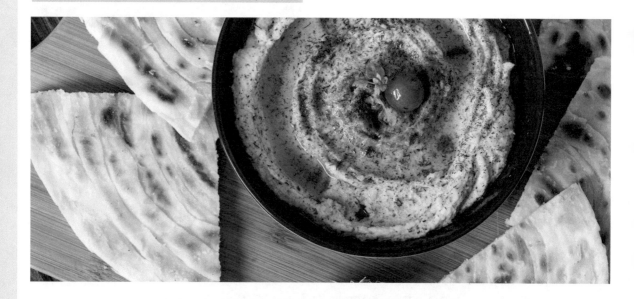

NUTRITIONAL INFORMATION

Calories 416, Fat 8.2g, Carbs 60.4g, Protein 25.8g

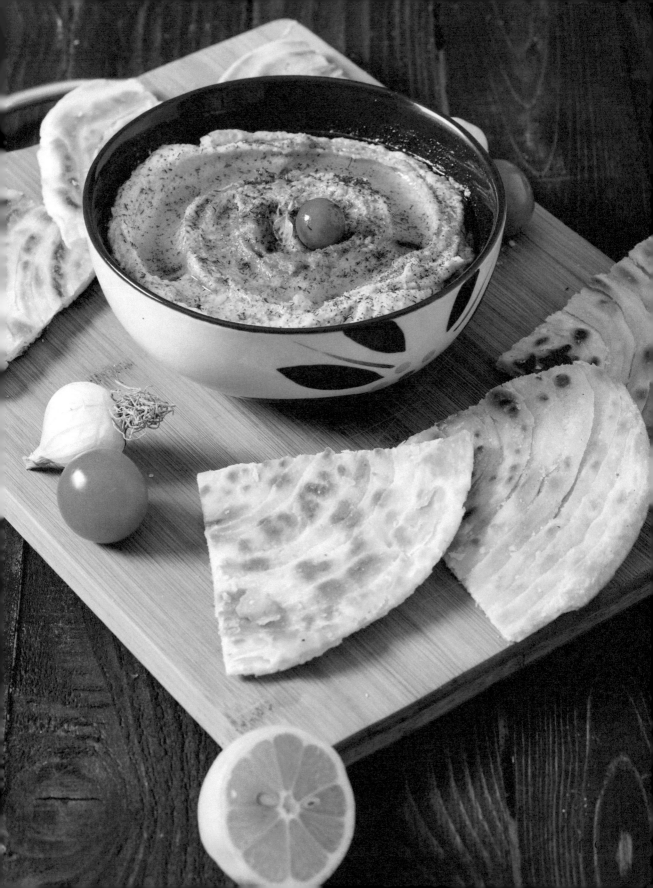

ROSEMARY AND SWEET POTATO CHIPS

 Cooking Difficulty: 2/10

 Cooking Time: 12 minutes

 Servings: 2

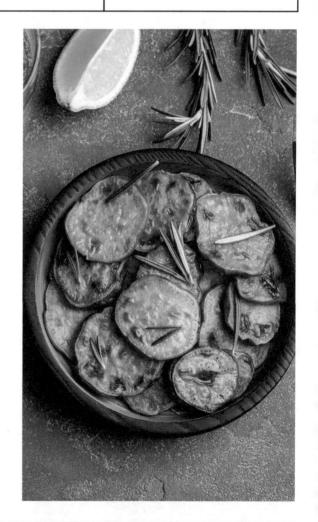

INGREDIENTS

- 1 tbsp. melted coconut oil
- 1 tsp. himalayan pink salt
- 2 large sweet potatoes
- 2 tsps. dried rosemary

NUTRITIONAL INFORMATION

90 Calories, 13g Carbs, 1g Protein, 3.5g Fat

DESCRIPTION

STEP 1
Preheat your oven to 375 degrees Fahrenheit.

STEP 2
Thinly slice the sweet potatoes using a mandolin.

STEP 3
Grind rosemary and Himalayan pink salt using mortar and pestle.

STEP 4
Place sweet potatoes in a bowl and add the salt-seasoning mixture and coconut oil.

STEP 5
Pour into a nonstick baking sheet and place it in the oven. After ten minutes, take the dish out and flip the chips.

STEP 6
Return it back to the oven and bake for another ten minutes.

STEP 7
Take the pan out of the oven and place the chips that are starting to brown in the cooling rack.

STEP 8
Return it back to the oven and bake for another 3 to 5 mins.

STEP 9
Once done, place all the chips in the cooling rack.

RAINBOW FRUIT SALAD

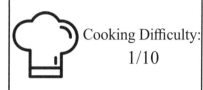 Cooking Difficulty: 1/10

 Cooking Time: 5 minutes

 Servings: 4

INGREDIENTS

for the fruit salad:
- 1 lb. hulled strawberries, sliced
- 1 c. kiwis, halved, cubed
- 1 ¼ c. blueberries
- 1 1/3 c. blackberries
- 1 c. pineapple chunks

for the maple lime dressing:
- 2 tsps. lime zest
- ¼ c. maple syrup
- 1 tbsp. lime juice

DESCRIPTION

STEP 1
Prepare the salad, and for this, take a bowl, place all its ingredients and toss until mixed.

STEP 2
Prepare the dressing, and for this, take a small bowl, place all its ingredients and whisk well.

STEP 3
Drizzle the dressing over salad, toss until coated and serve.

NUTRITIONAL INFORMATION

Calories: 88.1, Fat: 0.4 g, Carbs: 22.6 g, Protein: 1.1 g

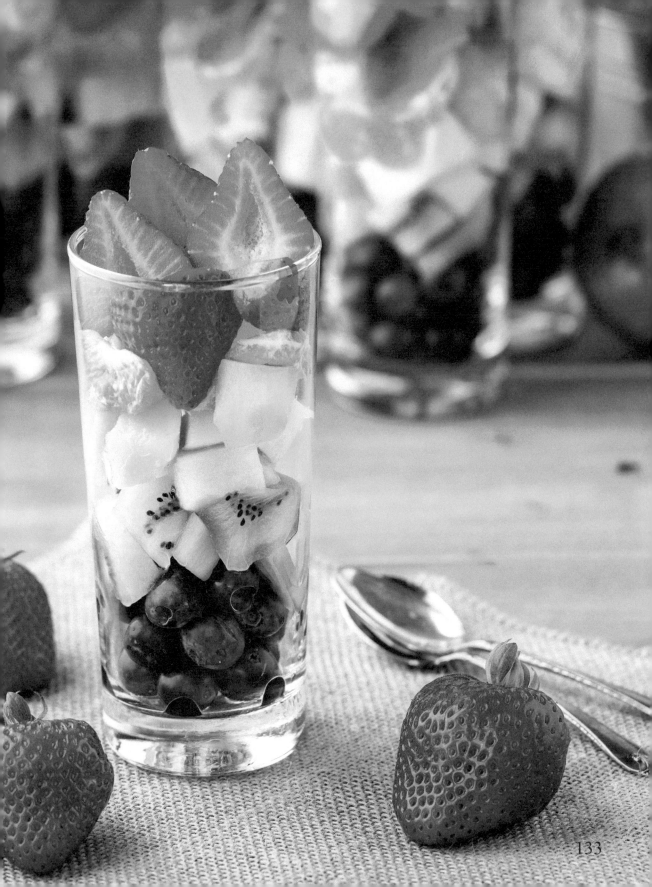

ALMONDS AND SEEDS BOWLS

 Cooking Difficulty: 1/10

 Cooking Time: 11 minutes

 Servings: 4

INGREDIENTS

- 1 c. sunflower seeds
- ¼ c. coconut, shredded
- cooking spray
- 2 c. almonds
- 1 mango, peeled and cubed
- hazelnuts and cashews if desired

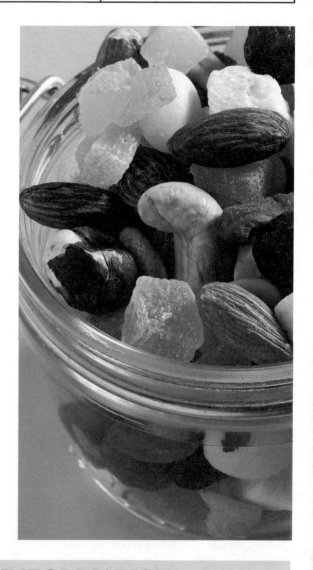

DESCRIPTION

STEP 1

Spread the almonds, coconut, mango, and sunflower seeds on a baking tray, grease with the cooking spray, toss and bake at 400 degrees F for 10 minutes. Divide into bowls and serve as a snack.

NUTRITIONAL INFORMATION

Calories 430, Fat 18.1g, Carbs 54g, Protein 14.5g

ROASTED WALNUTS

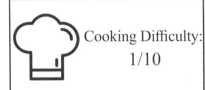 Cooking Difficulty: 1/10

 Cooking Time: 15 minutes

 Servings: 8

INGREDIENTS

- 14 oz. walnuts
- ½ tsp. garlic powder
- 1 tbsp. avocado oil
- ½ tsp. chili powder
- ½ tsp. smoked paprika
- ¼ tsp. cayenne pepper

DESCRIPTION

STEP 1

Spread the walnuts on a lined baking sheet, add the paprika and the other ingredients, toss and bake at 410 degrees F for 15 minutes. Divide into bowls and serve as a snack.

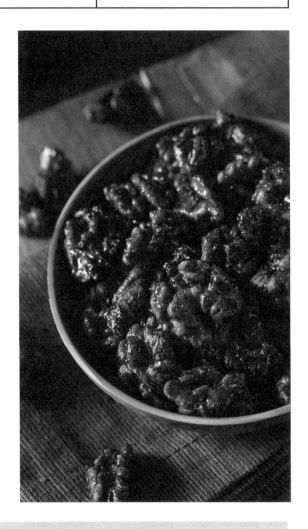

NUTRITIONAL INFORMATION

Calories 311, Fat 29.6g, Carbs 5.3g, Protein 12g

CRANBERRY SQUARES

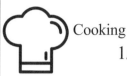 Cooking Difficulty: 1/10

 Cooking Time: 4 minutes

 Servings: 4

INGREDIENTS

- 2 tbsps. coconut, shredded
- 2 tbsps. rolled oats
- 1 c. cranberries
- 2 oz. coconut cream

DESCRIPTION

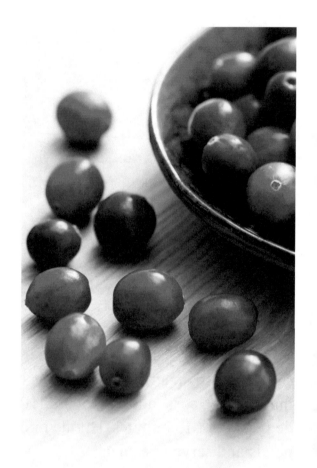

STEP 1

In a blender, combine the oats with the cranberries and the other ingredients, pulse well, and spread into a square pan.

STEP 2

Cut into squares and keep them in the fridge for 3 hours before serving.

NUTRITIONAL INFORMATION

Calories 32, Fat 0.7g, Carbs 6.1g, Protein 1.1g

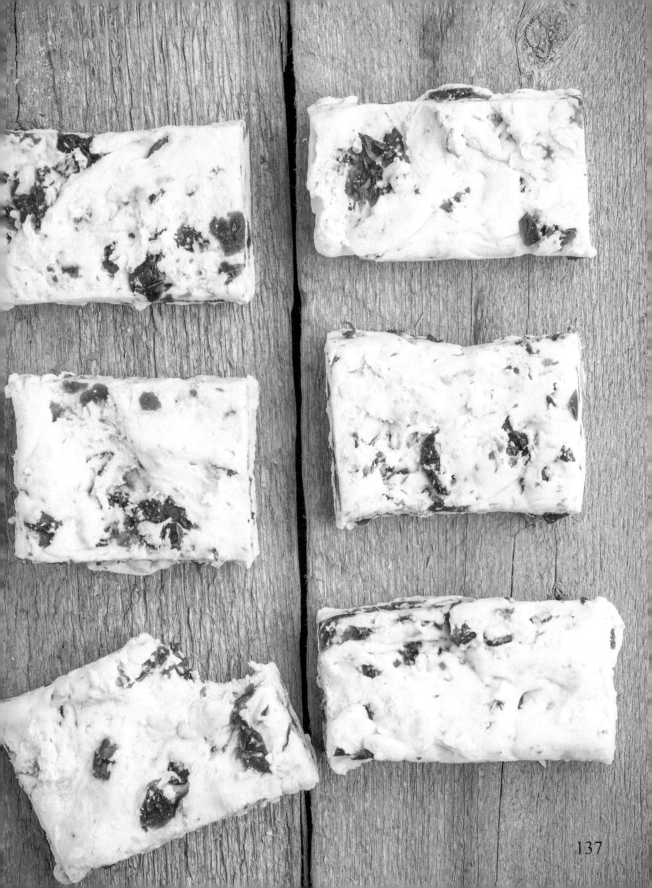

CONCLUSION

Every individual, regardless of their background, faces the potential risk of developing Alzheimer's disease and dementia. Factors such as family history, age, unhealthy dietary habits, sedentary lifestyles, high cholesterol, and smoking can contribute to an increased susceptibility.

Initiating positive changes for your health is a proactive step that can never start too early. Embracing the principles of the MIND diet stands as the foundation for minimizing risk and supplying your body and brain with essential nutrients. Incorporating fresh vegetables, fruits, nuts, olive oil, fish, and poultry into your weekly menu is a significant initial stride towards transformation.

In tandem with a nutritious diet, regular exercise is crucial. Begin with simple activities like a ten-minute walk, gradually incorporating a mix of cardio and strength training to maintain your weight and ensure optimal brain health.

A fulfilling lifestyle involves meaningful social interactions with friends, recognizing the innate social nature of human beings. Learning something new every day contributes to mental stimulation, a key pillar among the seven highlighted in this book. The holistic approach, encompassing a balanced diet, quality sleep, stress reduction, physical activity, social engagement, vascular health maintenance, and continuous mental stimulation, significantly reduces the risk of Alzheimer's.

I trust that this book has equipped you with essential insights to safeguard your brain's well-being. While we all confront the potential threat of Alzheimer's, your dedication to the seven pillars and the wholesome MIND diet will yield substantial benefits.

In closing, I express my gratitude for your readership. Adhere to the recommended diet, prioritize an active and social lifestyle, alleviate stress, and immerse yourself in activities you love, surrounded by those who bring joy and love into your life. May your journey towards optimal brain health be both rewarding and fulfilling.

Olivia Wood

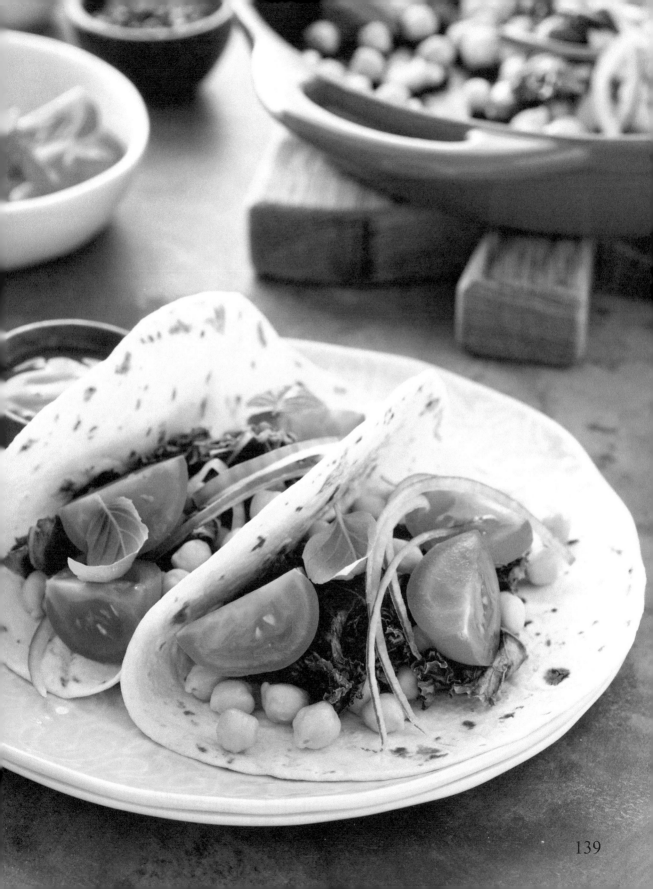

Made in United States
Troutdale, OR
12/06/2024

26003595R00077